# RevMED

## 400 SBAs in
## Preclinical Medicine

**Other Related Titles from World Scientific**

---

*RevMED 300 SBAs in Clinical Specialties*
by Lasith Ranasinghe and Oliver Clements
ISBN: 978-1-78634-846-3
ISBN: 978-1-78634-852-4 (pbk)

*RevMED 300 SBAs in Medicine and Surgery*
by Lasith Ranasinghe and Oliver Clements
ISBN: 978-1-78634-681-0
ISBN: 978-1-78634-711-4 (pbk)

*300 Single Best Answers in Clinical Medicine*
by George Collins, James Davis and Oscar Swift
edited by Huw Beynon
ISBN: 978-1-78326-436-0
ISBN: 978-1-78326-437-7 (pbk)

*320 Single Best Answer Questions for Final Year Medical Students*
*Second Edition*
by Adam Ioannou
ISBN: 978-981-121-008-2
ISBN: 978-981-121-077-8 (pbk)

*The PICU Book: A Primer for Medical Students, Residents and Acute*
*Care Practitioners*
edited by Ronald M Perkin, Irma Fiordalisi and William E Novotny
ISBN: 978-981-4329-60-6

*Surgical Talk: Lecture Notes in Undergraduate Surgery*
*Third Edition*
by Andrew Goldberg and Gerard Stansby
ISBN: 978-1-84816-614-1 (pbk)

# RevMED

## 400 SBAs in
## Preclinical Medicine

Lasith Ranasinghe • Harroop Bola

*Imperial College London, UK*

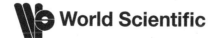 **World Scientific**

NEW JERSEY · LONDON · SINGAPORE · BEIJING · SHANGHAI · HONG KONG · TAIPEI · CHENNAI · TOKYO

*Published by*

World Scientific Publishing Europe Ltd.

57 Shelton Street, Covent Garden, London WC2H 9HE

*Head office:* 5 Toh Tuck Link, Singapore 596224

*USA office:* 27 Warren Street, Suite 401-402, Hackensack, NJ 07601

**Library of Congress Cataloging-in-Publication Data**
Names: Ranasinghe, Lasith, author. | Bola, Harroop, author.
Title: RevMED 400 SBAs in preclinical medicine / Lasith Ranasinghe, Harroop Bola.
Other titles: 400 SBAs in preclinical medicine
Description: New Jersey : World Scientific, [2022] | Includes index.
Identifiers: LCCN 2021027271 (print) | LCCN 2021027272 (ebook) |
    ISBN 9781800610712 (hardcover) | ISBN 9781800610873 (paperback) |
    ISBN 9781800610729 (ebook for institutions) | ISBN 9781800610736 (ebook for individuals)
Subjects: MESH: Physiological Phenomena | Genetic Phenomena |
    Cell Physiological Phenomena | Examination Questions
Classification: LCC QP40 (print) | LCC QP40 (ebook) | NLM QT 18.2 | DDC 612.0076--dc23
LC record available at https://lccn.loc.gov/2021027271
LC ebook record available at https://lccn.loc.gov/2021027272

**British Library Cataloguing-in-Publication Data**
A catalogue record for this book is available from the British Library.

For any available supplementary material, please visit
https://www.worldscientific.com/worldscibooks/10.1142/Q0316#t=suppl

Desk Editors: Aanand Jayaraman/Michael Beale/Shi Ying Koe

Typeset by Stallion Press
Email: enquiries@stallionpress.com

Printed in Singapore

# Foreword

Having taught thousands of pre-clinical medical students over the last decade, one aspect that has consistently remained difficult for students is retaining the sheer volume of factual knowledge that is required. Although, many people will have said this before me, I would reiterate that one of the more effective ways of learning for the knowledge-recall assessments is to regularly test yourself using targeted practice assessments.

As tutors, we try to put together as much formative assessment as possible, but this is something that you cannot get enough of! Dr. Lasith Ranasinghe was a multi-award-winning student and an active member of the student union during his MBBS degree. With the guidance of current MBBS students, he has produced this huge resource of targeted formative assessment questions, which will allow current students to supplement their active learning strategies and lead to successful outcomes!

Dr. Sohag Saleh
*Principal Teaching Fellow & Digital Development Lead*
*Imperial College School of Medicine*

# Preface

Every budding doctor will have experienced that feeling of intense excitement on their first day as a medical student. Though the volume of knowledge that lies ahead may seem daunting, it is overshadowed by the momentous end goal of becoming a fully-fledged doctor. It is important, nonetheless, to enjoy the journey and to avoid being in too much of a rush to get to the finishing line. This is particularly true during the preclinical years.

It may come as a surprise that the idea to write this preclinical book occurred to me only after starting work as a junior doctor in the NHS. It was inspired by the realisation that every patient that I see and every disease that I encounter is underpinned by the principles that I learnt during my preclinical years. Many students may, at times, struggle to see how some of the minutiae of biochemistry and physiology that they struggle through is relevant to their future lives as doctors. During these moments, I urge you to have faith in the system. The knowledge that you accumulate during these preclinical years will not only make you better at your job, but it will also make life as a doctor far more fascinating.

Dr. Lasith Ranasinghe
*RevMED Series*

# About the Authors

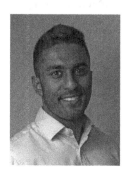 **Lasith Ranasinghe** is an Academic Foundation Doctor working at Imperial College Healthcare NHS Trust. He grew up in Norwich before moving to London to study medicine at Imperial College London in 2014. During his time at Imperial, he developed a reputation for producing outstanding medical educational resources and delivering regular teaching for his peers. He went on to co-chair the Medical Education (MedED) society and undertake the role of Academic Officer on the Students' Union. He maintained an exceptional academic standard throughout his time at medical school, winning 23 prizes for academic excellence and frequently ranking within the top 10 of his cohort. He has also started a medical education charity, *Make a Medic*, which runs courses for medical students and uses the funds raised to support medical education initiatives in developing countries, such as filling libraries and funding training programmes.

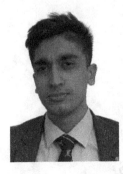

**Harroop Bola** is a medical student at Imperial College London. He grew up in Leicester before moving to London to study medicine. In 2020, he co-founded the British Indian Medical Association (BIMA) — a national organisation that aims to deliver a comprehensive medical education syllabus and improve access to peer-to-peer support. BIMA has developed a formidable, interconnected network of medical students and doctors, providing a wealth of opportunities both socially and professionally. He has also chaired the Imperial College Medical Education (MedED) society's online SBA platform, helped arrange mock examinations and disseminate academic resources amongst preclinical students. In the future, he hopes to pursue his interest in cardiothoracics with teaching being a prominent part of his career.

# List of Contributors

**Dr. Oliver Clements** — Brighton and Sussex University Hospitals
NHS Trust

**Chelsea Stubbs** — Imperial College London

**Virensinh Rathod** — Imperial College London

**Pratheeshan Sabeshan** — Imperial College London

**Zain Islam** — Imperial College London

**Varja Čučulović** — Imperial College London

**Ashwin Venkatakrishnan** — Imperial College London

# Contents

# Part 1

# Basic Sciences for Medicine

# Cells and Metabolism

## Questions

1. How is the rate of glycolysis controlled within the cytoplasm of a cell?

   A Glucose-6-phosphate directly inhibits hexokinase activity

   B Pyruvate saturation within the cytoplasm reduces pyruvate kinase activity

   C Phosphoglucose isomerase is allosterically controlled by ATP

   D ATP exerts an inhibitory effect on phosphofructokinase activity

   E The rate is controlled by the available concentration of oxaloacetate

2. In what form is cholesterol transported after being absorbed within the small intestine?

   A Chylomicrons

   B High-density lipoproteins

   C Low-density lipoproteins

   D Very low-density lipoproteins

   E Intermediate density lipoproteins

3. What type of necrosis is associated with acute pancreatitis?

    **A** Coagulative necrosis
    **B** Caseous necrosis
    **C** Liquefactive necrosis
    **D** Fat necrosis
    **E** Necroptosis

4. A 61-year-old man is recovering on the cardiology ward after having an ST-elevation myocardial infarction. He has been discharged on a number of medications, including atorvastatin (statin).
Given the mechanism of action of this drug, which substrate is directly affected?

    **A** Squalene
    **B** Mevalonate
    **C** Farnesyl pyrophosphate
    **D** Lanosterol
    **E** Cholesterol

5. Which of the following cell-cell connections is crucial to the mechanical stability of a layer of cells?

    **A** Tight junctions
    **B** Adherens junction
    **C** Gap junction
    **D** Desmosomes
    **E** Connexons

6. A 74-year-old patient has had a biopsy taken from his bronchus after presenting with haemoptysis. The epithelium appears multilayered, with all apical cells maintaining contact with the basal lamina.
Which type of epithelium has been described?

    **A** Simple columnar epithelium
    **B** Simple squamous epithelium

**C** Stratified squamous epithelium
**D** Stratified cuboidal epithelium
**E** Pseudostratified epithelium

7. Which of the following enzymes is often measured in the diagnosis of a myocardial infarction?

    **A** Hexokinase IV
    **B** Pyruvate dehydrogenase
    **C** Lactate dehydrogenase
    **D** Creatine kinase
    **E** Troponin

8. Which of the following best describes the mechanism of action of rotenone?

    **A** Inhibits the transfer of electrons from complex I to ubiquinone
    **B** Binds onto the stalk of ATP synthase and inhibits oxidative phosphorylation
    **C** Inhibits pyruvate dehydrogenase activity
    **D** Inhibits cytochrome oxidase activity
    **E** Uncouples oxidative phosphorylation from ATP production by providing an alternate route for proton flow

9. Which vitamin deficiency causes beriberi?

    **A** Thiamine
    **B** Folate
    **C** Vitamin B2
    **D** Vitamin B12
    **E** Vitamin D

10. Which family of proteins is responsible for regulating the sequential progression of the various stages of the cell cycle?

    **A** BUB kinases
    **B** Centromere Protein-E
    **C** Cyclins
    **D** RAF kinases
    **E** Mitogens

11. Which of the following is an example of autocrine signalling?

    **A** Action of glucagon on pancreatic beta cells
    **B** Production of osteoclast-activating factors by osteoblasts
    **C** Action of IL2 on activated T lymphocytes
    **D** T-cell receptor interaction with an MHC Class II molecule
    **E** HIV GP120 interacting with a CD4 receptor

12. A 42-year-old woman visits her GP after noticing a lump in her neck. On examination, there is a firm lump in the right lobe of the thyroid gland. She is concerned about the lump being cancerous and would like to have it investigated further.
    Which of the following investigations is most appropriate in this case?

    **A** Core biopsy
    **B** Frozen section
    **C** Resection specimen
    **D** Fine needle aspiration
    **E** Trephine biopsy

13. Which of the following is an ionotropic receptor?

    **A** AT1 angiotensin receptor
    **B** M2 muscarinic receptor
    **C** Nicotinic acetylcholine receptor
    **D** $\beta_1$ adrenergic receptor
    **E** H1 histamine receptor

14. Which of these Krebs cycle enzymes is found on the inner surface of the mitochondrial membrane?

A Fumarase
B Succinate dehydrogenase
C Malate dehydrogenase
D Citrate synthase
E α-ketoglutarate dehydrogenase

15. A 32-year-old patient is diagnosed with COPD after becoming increasingly breathless with reduced exercise tolerance over the past 6 months. He was also recently diagnosed with cirrhosis after becoming jaundiced and coagulopathic.
A deficiency of which of the following proteins would explain his clinical state?

    A Albumin
    B $\alpha_1$-antitrypsin
    C Haptoglobin
    D Complement
    E Gamma globulins

16. Vinblastine is a mitotic spindle poison used in the treatment of Hodgkin lymphoma. It interferes with tubulin within the spindle microtubules and prevents the splitting of chromosomes into sister chromatids. During which stage of mitosis are the chromosomes separated?

    A Prophase
    B Prometaphase
    C Metaphase
    D Anaphase
    E Telophase

17. Which ATP synthase F0 subunit initially rotates due to the passive flow of protons from the intermembrane space?

    A B subunit
    B C subunit
    C Beta subunit

    **D** Gamma subunit

    **E** Alpha subunit

18. Which enzyme is activated as part of a response to hyperglycemic conditions?

    **A** Adipose lipoprotein lipase
    **B** Adipose triglyceride lipase
    **C** Glucose-6-phosphatase
    **D** Dipeptidyl peptidase 4
    **E** GLUT2

19. How does cytosolic NADH transfer electrons to the mitochondria?

    **A** NADH reduces dihydroxyacetone phosphate to glycerol-3-phosphate under the action of mitochondrial enzymes
    **B** NADH transfers electrons using the glycerol-phosphate shuttle, initially reducing cytosolic glycerol-3-phosphate
    **C** NADH reduces cytosolic oxaloacetate to malate, crossing into the inner mitochondrial membrane
    **D** NADH reduces cytosolic aspartate to oxaloacetate, crossing into the inner mitochondrial membrane
    **E** NADH directly transfers electrons to mitochondrial FAD

20. A group of neutrophils exhibit morphological changes including nuclear shrinkage (pyknosis) and fragmentation (karyorrhexis) after an acute inflammatory response.
    Which cell process is occurring?

    **A** Necrosis
    **B** Apoptosis
    **C** Necroptosis
    **D** NETosis
    **E** Entosis

21. Which metabolic pathway is primarily affected in MCAD deficiency?

A  Glycolysis
B  Beta oxidation
C  Oxidative phosphorylation
D  Krebs cycle
E  Lipogenesis

22. How is hexokinase I adapted to perform its metabolic role effectively?

A  Low glucose affinity
B  High Michaelis constant
C  High $V_{max}$
D  Regulated by glucose-6-phosphatase activity
E  Sensitive to negative feedback from glucose-6-phosphate

23. A 61-year-old man has been diagnosed with osteoarthritis affecting both of his knees.
Which proteoglycan is predominantly affected in osteoarthritis?

A  Aggrecan
B  Type I collagen
C  Decorin
D  Perlecan
E  Syndecan

24. Aneuploidy occurs due to defects in the mitotic spindle checkpoint.
Which stage of mitosis is delayed during this checkpoint?

A  Prophase
B  Prometaphase
C  Metaphase
D  Anaphase
E  Telophase

25. A 23-year-old patient with a background of nephrotic syndrome has been admitted with severe generalised oedema. He is treated with IV human albumin solution.

Which of the following factors is responsible for his generalised oedema?

A  Increased plasma oncotic pressure
B  Decreased plasma oncotic pressure
C  Increased hydrostatic pressure
D  Decreased hydrostatic pressure
E  Increased capillary permeability

26. During glycolysis, the phosphoryl group in glycerate-3-phosphate shifts to form 2-phosphoglycerate.
What type of reaction is this an example of?

A  Group transfer reaction
B  Hydrolytic reaction
C  Oxidation-reduction reaction
D  Isomerisation reaction
E  Ligation reaction requiring ATP cleavage

27. What is the cellular target of oligomycin?

A  ATP synthase
B  Complex I
C  Complex II
D  Cytochrome oxidase
E  Coenzyme Q

28. Which of the following best describes the function of a centromere?

A  Forms the microtubule organising centre
B  Chromatid adhesion and segregation
C  Dissolves nuclear envelope
D  Chromosome condensation
E  Initiates cytokinesis

29. Palmitic acid is a 16-carbon saturated fatty acid sourced from palm oils.

    What is the maximal yield of ATP molecules that can be generated given palmitic acid undergoes complete beta oxidation?

    A 128
    B 129
    C 131
    D 134
    E 136

30. The Krebs cycle is a major component of aerobic respiration that results in the production of ATP.

    Which substrate within the Krebs cycle is converted to fumarate via the reduction of FAD?

    A Citrate
    B $\alpha$-ketoglutarate
    C Malate
    D Succinate
    E Oxaloacetate

## Answers

### 1. D (ATP exerts an inhibitory effect on phosphofructokinase activity)

The rate of glycolysis within cells is determined by ATP, which exerts an inhibitory effect on phosphofructokinase. As glycolysis proceeds, the cytoplasmic concentration of ATP will increase, thereby exerting a negative regulatory effect on glycolysis. Phosphofructokinase is an enzyme that plays an important role high up in the glycolysis pathway — it phosphorylates fructose-6-phosphate into fructose-1,6-bisphosphate.

Glucose-6-phosphate concentrations are dependent on phosphofructokinase activity. Pyruvate can be shunted via the anaerobic pathway to generate ATP via anaerobic respiration. Therefore, it does not limit glycolysis. Phosphoglucose isomerase is responsible for the isomerisation of glucose-6-phosphate into fructose-6-phosphate. It does not regulate glycolysis. Oxaloacetate is a primary substrate used in the Krebs cycle. This process happens within the mitochondria, not the cytoplasm.

### 2. A (Chylomicrons)

Fats from the diet are absorbed by the enterocytes lining the brush border of the small intestine and are reformed into triglycerides within the endoplasmic reticulum. They will then be packaged into large particles called chylomicrons. These are absorbed into the lymphatics and will eventually enter the systemic circulation. Lipoprotein lipase, found within the endothelial cells lining adipose tissue, cardiac and skeletal muscle, will hydrolyse the triglycerides within the chylomicrons into fatty acids and glycerol. Chylomicrons can also acquire apoproteins from high-density lipoproteins (HDLs) which transform them into low-density lipoproteins (LDLs) and very low-density lipoproteins (VLDLs).

HDLs are synthesised within the liver and are associated with a reduced risk of cardiovascular disease. LDLs are the dangerous forms of cholesterol that are able to enter the arterial intima resulting in the formation of atherosclerotic deposits. VLDLs are synthesised in the liver and transfer triglycerides and cholesterol to both adipose and muscle tissue. Intermediate density lipoproteins (IDLs) are LDL precursors.

### 3. D (Fat necrosis)

Acute pancreatitis is a condition in which the pancreas becomes inflamed resulting in acinar injury. The most common causes of acute pancreatitis are gallstones and alcohol excess, which both result in the premature activation of enzymes within the pancreas, resulting in autodigestion. The action of lipases can result in the breakdown of fats within the pancreas giving rise to the histological appearance of fat necrosis. Furthermore, lipases can break down triglycerides to release free fatty acids which can bind to calcium in a process called saponification. It can result in hypocalcaemia.

Coagulative necrosis is a form of tissue death resulting from ischaemia. The connective tissue architecture may remain intact whilst the cells in between die. Myocardial infarction is an example of coagulative necrosis. Caseous necrosis is a form of tissue death that occurs in the lungs, usually due to tuberculosis. Liquefactive necrosis is a process by which tissue death results in the formation of a fluid-filled space. This most commonly occurs in the brain. Necroptosis is a form of cell death that demonstrates features of both necrosis and apoptosis.

### 4. B (Mevalonate)

Statins are medications that are commonly used in the treatment of hypercholesterolaemia. It may also be used as part of secondary prevention in patients who have had a myocardial infarction or stroke. Statins work by inhibiting HMG-CoA reductase which is an important enzyme in cholesterol metabolism. It converts mevalonate into HMG-CoA which is an early step in the cholesterol synthesis pathway.

### 5. D (Desmosomes)

Desmosomes are a form of cell-cell connection that have an anchoring effect on a line of cells. It provides mechanical stability due to its strong adhesive effect. This enables cells to have polarity.

Tight junctions may be found between the apical and lateral membranes of adjacent cells. As the name suggests, it forms very tight connections between the cells that regulated the passage of molecules via the paracellular route. Adherens junctions provide the stabilisation and initiation of cell-cell adhesion by regulating the actin cytoskeleton and holding adjacent epithelial cells together. Gap junctions (channel-forming) facilitate the movement of molecules and ions between cells. They are composed of two connexons (hemichannels). Gap junctions enable electrical communication between cells (e.g. the electrical activity of the heart). Connexons are the components that form a gap junction.

## 6. E (Pseudostratified epithelium)

Pseudostratified epithelium appears to have several layers; however, all apical cells have some contact with the basal lamina. It is predominantly found within the respiratory tract (trachea and bronchi), urinary tract and reproductive tract.

Simple columnar epithelium describes a single layer of columnar cells. It is mainly found in the gastrointestinal tract. Simple squamous epithelium is a single layer of flat cells. The endothelium lining the circulatory system is a form of simple squamous epithelium. Stratified squamous epithelium is formed by multiple layers of flat cells. It can be described as keratinising or non-keratinising depending on whether they have a thick layer of keratin. The skin is an example of keratinising stratified squamous epithelium. The oesophagus is an example of non-keratinising stratified squamous epithelium. Stratified cuboidal epithelium is formed by several layers of cuboidal cells. It is found lining the ducts of sweat glands, salivary glands and mammary glands.

## 7. E (Troponin)

Troponins are enzymes that are important in muscle contraction. Troponin I and T are isoforms that are mainly found within cardiomyocytes. Damage to cardiomyocytes (e.g. in myocardial infarction) results in the leakage of troponins into the peripheral circulation, thereby giving a high value on the blood test. This is of huge diagnostic importance in suspected myocardial infarction.

Hexokinase IV is an intracellular enzyme responsible for the initial phosphorylation of glucose into glucose-6-phosphate during glycolysis. Pyruvate dehydrogenase converts pyruvate into acetyl-CoA. Lactate dehydrogenase (LDH) is an intracellular enzyme that is found in a variety of tissues across the body. As it is so widespread, a raised LDH is not very specific and can arise due to a number of causes, including tissue infarction, haemolysis and cancers. Creatine kinase (CK) is an enzyme that is found in muscle. A high creatine kinase can be suggestive of muscle damage (e.g. rhabdomyolysis following a fall and long lie). There are three main isoforms of creatine kinase: MM (skeletal muscle), BB (brain) and MB (heart). Although CK-MB is mainly found within the heart, troponins are favoured as a marker of infarction.

## 8. A (Inhibits the transfer of electrons from complex I to ubiquinone)

Rotenone is a chemical found in the roots and seeds of some plants. It inhibits the transfer of electrons from complex I to ubiquinone. This results in a blockage of electron flow down the electron transport chain.

Oligomycin is an antibiotic produced by streptomyces, which inhibits oxidative phosphorylation by binding to the F0 subunit of ATP synthase. This results in the accumulation of protons in the intermembrane space of the mitochondrion. Saturation of the intermembrane space reduces the capacity of protons to be actively pumped out, thus inhibiting electron flow in the electron transport chain. Arsenic inhibits pyruvate dehydrogenase, which results in a reduced conversion of pyruvate into acetyl-CoA. This is an essential substrate that enters the Krebs cycle and generates ATP. Cytochrome oxidase is the main target of cyanide poisoning. Cyanide binds irreversibly to the haem group within cytochrome oxidase, thereby preventing the final electron transfer step within the electron transport chain. Dinitrophenol is a compound that uncouples oxidative phosphorylation from ATP synthesis thereby increasing the body's metabolic rate. It has, due to this mechanism, been marketed illegally as a weight loss agent.

## 9. A (Thiamine)

Beriberi is a clinical syndrome caused by thiamine (vitamin B1) deficiency. Thiamine plays an important role in carbohydrate metabolism and a deficiency of thiamine results in widespread peripheral nervous system damage, muscle weakness and heart failure.

Folate deficiency and vitamin B12 deficiency are associated with megaloblastic anaemia. Vitamin B12 is also required for the myelination of neurones, and deficiency can result in peripheral neuropathy. Vitamin B2 is required for carbohydrate metabolism and has a role in maintaining the integrity of the skin, eyes and nervous system. Vitamin D is a major factor in calcium homeostasis. It increases intestinal absorption of calcium and reduces renal excretion. Deficiency can result in rickets (in children) or osteomalacia (in adults).

## 10. C (Cyclins)

Cyclins are transiently expressed at specific points in the cell cycle. They activate cyclin-dependent kinases (CDKs) which can phosphorylate and, hence, activate target proteins that promote progression of the cell cycle. The sequential activation of CDKs will stimulate genes at necessary intervals to allow the cell cycle to progress.

BUB kinases bind to the kinetochore fibres and dissociate once the chromosomes are appropriately attached to a spindle. They play a crucial role in the spindle assembly checkpoint. Centromere Protein-E (CENP-E) binds to kinetochore fibres and regulates chromosome motility. RAF kinases are serine/threonine protein kinases that are involved in cell signalling. Mitogens are a group of proteins that provide a signal to cells to undergo mitosis by inducing the expression of various proteins that are involved in regulating the cell cycle (e.g. cyclins).

## 11.  C (Action of IL2 on activated T lymphocytes)

Autocrine signalling is a form of cell signalling and hormone regulation by which the secreted hormone binds to receptors found on the cell that produced the hormone, thereby inducing a change in cell activity. The activation of T-cells will result in a cascade of intracellular events that results in an increased expression of interleukin 2 (IL2). The IL2 secreted by the T-cell will bind onto the IL2 receptor on the same T-cell, thereby stimulating the differentiation of the activated T-cell into effector T-cells and memory T-cells.

The effect of glucagon, which is produced by the alpha cells of the pancreas, on the beta cells is considered a form of paracrine signalling as it is acting in the local vicinity of the cells that produced it. Osteoclast activating factors are secreted by osteoblasts and have an effect on osteoclasts. This is also a form of paracrine signalling. GP120 interaction with the CD4 receptor is another form of membrane protein interaction.

## 12.  D (Fine needle aspiration)

Fine needle aspiration (FNA) is a type of biopsy specimen in which a needle is inserted into a lump to collect a sample of cells. It is often used in thyroid lumps. The sample will be sent for cytological analysis which can help determine whether a lump is benign or malignant.

A core biopsy is a similar technique in which a slightly larger needle is used such that a larger sample of tissue with its architecture can be obtained. This can be sent for histological analysis and tumour grading. Core biopsies are used in the diagnostic work-up of breast lumps. A frozen section is a technique used during surgical procedures in which samples can be rapidly sent to the pathology lab for analysis by a histopathologist. They, therefore, allow rapid identification of tissue and feedback to the surgeons in case a wider resection margin is required. During an operation, a sample of tissue can be removed and sent for histopathological analysis (e.g. left hemicolectomy for left-sided colorectal cancer). The outcome of histological analysis may guide ongoing treatment following completion of the surgical intervention. A trephine biopsy is used to sample bone marrow.

### 13. C (Nicotinic acetylcholine receptor)

Ionotropic receptors are membrane-bound receptor proteins that respond to ligand binding by opening an ion channel, thereby allowing the flow of ions through the cell membrane.

AT1 angiotensin receptors and H1 histamine receptors are examples of Gq receptors which work by stimulating phospholipase C. M2 muscarinic receptors are $G_i$ receptors which work by inhibiting adenylyl cyclase. $\beta_1$ adrenergic receptors are $G_s$ receptors which work by stimulating adenylyl cyclase.

### 14. B (Succinate dehydrogenase)

Succinate dehydrogenase is an enzyme associated with complex II, responsible for catalysing the oxidation of succinate to fumarate. FAD is the hydrogen carrier involved in this oxidation step, whereby it becomes reduced to FADH2 after accepting a pair of electrons from succinate. FADH2 will become re-oxidised into FAD by transferring electrons to iron sulphide proteins in complex II.

Fumarase converts fumarate to malate and is found within the mitochondrial matrix. Malate dehydrogenase converts malate to oxaloacetate and is found within the mitochondrial matrix. Citrate synthase converts oxaloacetate to citrate and is found in the mitochondrial matrix. $\alpha$-ketoglutarate dehydrogenase converts $\alpha$-ketoglutarate to succinyl-CoA and is found in the mitochondrial matrix.

### 15. B ($\alpha_1$-antitrypsin)

Neutrophil elastase is a protease that is released by activated neutrophils and macrophages to break down pathogens and damaged host tissue.

These proteases are capable of causing considerable collateral damage when released into inflamed tissues, so neutrophil elastase inhibitors are essential in preventing unwanted damage to surrounding tissues. $\alpha_1$-antitrypsin deficiency is an inherited condition in which patients are unable to produce sufficient quantities of functional $\alpha_1$-antitrypsin. This results in an increased risk of protease-mediated damage, particularly in the liver and lungs. It typically manifests with early-onset COPD and cirrhosis.

Albumin is synthesised within the liver and plays an important role in hormone transport and the maintenance of intravascular volume. Chronic liver disease leads to oedema due to a reduction in hepatic albumin production. Haptoglobin is a member of the $\alpha_2$ globulin family and is responsible for binding to haemoglobin released by red cells when they are broken down. The subsequent haptoglobin-haemoglobin complex is removed by the spleen. Haptoglobins have an important role in the diagnosis of haemolytic anaemia. The increase in red cell destruction leads to an increase in the consumption of haptoglobins, so a low haptoglobin level is suggestive of haemolytic anaemia. Complement proteins are part of an important mechanism that facilitates our immune response to infection. Deficiency would result in an increased risk of infection. Gammaglobulins include immunoglobulins which, if deficient, can lead to several different syndromes characterised by an increased risk of infection.

## 16.  D (Anaphase)

Vinblastine works by binding to tubulin proteins and preventing the assembly of microtubules. This means that the spindles are unable to bind to chromosomes, so the chromosomes cannot be separated. This occurs during anaphase.

During prophase, chromosome condensation occurs which reduces the possibility of fragmentation during mitosis. The chromosomes become visible as sister chromatids attached by a centromere. During prometaphase, centrosomes migrate to opposite ends of the nucleus and begin to organise microtubules that radiate towards the centromeres of the chromosomes. During metaphase, the chromosomes align themselves to the spindle equator. This stage cannot proceed in the presence of vinblastine due to the impairment in microtubule formation. Telophase is the final stage of mitosis, whereby a new nuclear envelope forms around each group of chromatids. This establishes two sister nuclei and prepares the cell for cytokinesis.

## 17.  B (C subunit)

ATP synthase is a multimeric enzyme consisting of a membrane-bound part (F0) and a part which projects into the matrix space (F1). F1 and F0 both consist of three distinct subunits, a, b & c, and alpha, beta and gamma, respectively. Protons will diffuse down the electrochemical gradient from the intermembrane space via the pore. This facilitates the rotation of the disc of C subunits. This passive movement of protons releases energy and causes a conformational change in ATP synthase. The gamma subunit of F1 is coupled with the disc and rotates simultaneously, however, the alpha and beta subunits do not rotate as the beta subunit is anchored to membrane subunit a. The rotation driven by proton movement leads to conformational changes in the protein which alters its affinity for ADP thereby resulting in the generation of ATP.

## 18.  A (Adipose lipoprotein lipase)

A rise in serum glucose concentration (usually due to the recent ingestion of carbohydrates) will result in the release of insulin from the pancreatic beta cells. Insulin will stimulate the mechanisms of storing glucose (e.g. glycogenesis, lipogenesis, proteogenesis) and inhibit mechanisms for releasing glucose (e.g. gluconeogenesis, glycogenolysis, lipolysis, proteolysis). Insulin also upregulates adipose lipoprotein lipase activity which is responsible for hydrolysing chylomicrons and facilitating the movement of fatty acids into adipose tissue where it can be stored.

Adipose triglyceride lipases break down adipose tissue into fatty acids and monoacylglycerols which can be used for beta oxidation. It is the first reaction of lipolysis. Hepatic glucose-6-phosphatase is important in the liberation of glucose from glucose-6-phosphate during glycogenolysis and gluconeogenesis. Insulin inhibits this enzyme. Dipeptidyl peptidase 4 (DPP4) is responsible for the breakdown of incretins, which are blood glucose-dependent hormones that can stimulate a reduction in serum glucose. DPP4 inhibitors are used in the treatment of diabetes mellitus as it can potentiate the incretin effect resulting in lower blood glucose levels. GLUT2 is the glucose transporter found in the beta cells of the pancreas and acts as the main glucose sensor of the pancreas.

## 19. D (NADH reduces cytosolic aspartate to oxaloacetate, crossing into the inner mitochondrial membrane)

Electrons from cytosolic NADH are transferred into the mitochondrion by the malate-aspartate shuttle. It is mediated by two membrane carriers and four enzymes. Oxaloacetate is reduced and electrons are gained from NADH to form malate via the action of malate dehydrogenase. Malate traverses the inner mitochondrial membrane and is re-oxidised by NAD+ in the matrix to form NADH and oxaloacetate. This oxaloacetate cannot cross the inner mitochondrial membrane so a transamination reaction is required to convert the oxaloacetate into aspartate before it can traverse the membrane. Within the cytosol, aspartate will be acted upon by a transaminase to produce glutamate and oxaloacetate. The inner mitochondrial membrane is relatively impermeable to NADH and NAD+, however, electrons from NADH are transferred via the mitochondrial membrane. This is mediated by the glycerol-phosphate shuttle.

## 20. B (Apoptosis)

Apoptosis is programmed cell death in response to stress. It is mediated by the timely activation of caspases that results in the degradation of cellular structures including the cytoskeleton and nucleus. This results in various morphological changes including pyknosis and karyorrhexis. Neutrophils are the first responders of the immune system and can be found in abundance in acutely inflamed tissue. Once they have carried out their role of phagocytosing pathogens and cellular debris, they will apoptose and then they, themselves, will be phagocytosed by macrophages.

Necrosis is confluent cell death in response to a pathological stress. Necrotic cell death is disorganised and results in the release of various cellular contents which triggers an inflammatory response. Necroptosis is a hybrid form of cell death that exhibits features of necrosis and apoptosis. It can be induced by viruses such as HIV. Neutrophil extracellular traps (NET) are networks of extracellular fibres that can bind and kill pathogens. They can also activate a suicide mechanism in which the neutrophils die via a process known as NETosis. Entosis is a process by which a living cell invades and becomes encapsulated by another cell's cytoplasm. This can trigger cell death.

### 21.  B (Beta oxidation)

Medium-chain acyl-CoA dehydrogenase (MCAD) deficiency is a rare autosomal recessive condition that, if left undiagnosed, can be fatal. A range of acyl-CoA dehydrogenases are responsible for catalysing the progressive breakdown of fatty acids via beta oxidation within the mitochondrial matrix. They are described based on the length of the fatty acids they process (e.g. short-, medium- and long-chain acyl CoA dehydrogenase). The acetyl-CoA molecules generated by beta oxidation can then enter the Krebs cycle to generate ATP and electron carriers for oxidative phosphorylation. This process is particularly important in providing an energy supply during fasted states in which glucose is in short supply. In MCAD deficiency, patients lack an enzyme that is required for beta oxidation. Therefore, their ability to generate a usable form of energy during fasted states is compromised. Patients with MCAD deficiency, therefore, should not fast for longer than 10–12 hours and, in particular, must have a constant supply of carbohydrates as they are unable to rely on beta oxidation.

### 22.  E (Sensitive to negative feedback from glucose-6-phosphate)

Hexokinase I is a glucokinase that is mainly found within muscle. It catalyses the initial phosphorylation of glucose to glucose-6-phosphate within the cell and is considered the rate-limiting step of glucose metabolism. It is regulated by a negative feedback loop in which a rise in glucose-6-phosphate concentration results in a reduction in hexokinase I.

Hexokinase I has a high affinity for glucose. The Michaelis constant is the concentration of substrate required for the enzyme to function at half its maximal rate. Hexokinase I in muscle has a Michaelis constant of 0.1 mM which suggests that the enzyme is active at low concentrations of glucose. $V_{max}$ is the maximal rate of enzyme action. Given the low Michaelis constant of hexokinase I, it operates at its maximum rate at relatively low glucose concentrations. It is not regulated by glucose-6-phosphatase activity.

## 23. A (Aggrecan)

Osteoarthritis is a disease of the cartilage that results in excessive degradation of the extracellular matrix. This compromises the ability of cartilaginous joints to lubricate joints and protect bones. Aggrecan is a major cartilaginous matrix component that is degraded by aggrecanases and metalloproteinases in osteoarthritis. Osteoarthritis may be caused by the presence of abnormal joint cartilage (i.e. some families are predisposed to developing osteoarthritis as their cartilage is more fragile) or abnormal joint forces (e.g. repetitive use in sportspeople or obesity).

Collagen is a major extracellular matrix protein that contributes to connective tissue throughout the body. There are five main types of collagen. Type I collagen is found in skin, tendons and bone. Type II collagen is found in articular cartilage. Decorin is a small leucine-rich proteoglycan involved in the regulation of the cell cycle. Perlecan is a heparan sulphate proteoglycan that is responsible for maintaining the stability of the basement membrane. It is also found within the endothelium. Syndecan is a cell surface proteoglycan that can act as a co-receptor for G-protein coupled receptors.

## 24. D (Anaphase)

The spindle assembly checkpoint monitors the status of chromosome-microtubule attachments and delays the onset of anaphase until all the kinetochores have formed stable bipolar connections to the mitotic spindle.

BUB kinases bind to kinetochore fibres and dissociate once chromosomes are securely attached to the spindle. This is a mechanism of quality controlling the connections formed. In aneuploidy, mis-attachment of microtubules to kinetochore fibres arises due to defects in the mitotic spindle checkpoint.

### 25.  B (Decreased plasma oncotic pressure)

Nephrotic syndrome is a condition in which large amounts of protein leaks into the urine, resulting in a hypoalbuminaemic state. As blood passes through capillary beds, fluid will leak out into the interstitium due to hydrostatic pressure. Much of this fluid will be drawn back into the circulation due to an oncotic pressure applied by large negatively charged proteins such as albumin. Any remaining fluid will return to the circulation via the lymphatics. The loss of large amounts of protein in the urine and the subsequent hypoalbuminaemic state will decrease the plasma oncotic pressure, thereby resulting in the accumulation of larger volumes of fluid within the interstitium. Albumin infusions may, therefore, be used as an intermediate measure to help the oedema resolve.

### 26.  D (Isomerisation reaction)

2-Phosphoglycerate is a positional isomer of glycerate-3-phosphate as the elemental composition of the molecule has not changed — a phosphoryl group has merely changed position. This is catalysed by phosphoglycerate mutase. Mutases are enzymes that catalyse the intramolecular shift of a chemical group.

### 27.  A (ATP synthase)

Oligomycin is an antibiotic produced by streptomyces. It inhibits oxidative phosphorylation by binding to the F0 subunit of ATP synthase. This inhibition blocks proton flow through the enzyme, thereby resulting in an accumulation of protons in the intermembrane space of the mitochondrion. Saturation of the intermembrane space reduces the capacity of protons to be actively pumped out, thereby inhibiting flow in the electron transport chain.

Complex I is the initial electron carrier within the transfer chain. After being reduced by NADH oxidation, it transfers electrons to coenzyme Q. Inhibition of complex I will decrease NADH oxidation and subsequent proton pumping across the inner mitochondrial membrane. This decreases the proton gradient between the inner mitochondrial membrane and inter-membrane space, thereby decreasing the rate of oxidative phosphoryla-tion. Rotenone is an agent that inhibits complex I. Malonate is an endogenous complex II inhibitor. It inhibits succinate dehydrogenase, thereby reducing electron flow from succinate to coenzyme Q along the electron transport chain. This, in turn, reduces the rate of oxidative phos-phorylation. Cytochrome oxidase is the main target of cyanide. It binds irreversibly to the haem group of cytochrome oxidase, thereby blocking the final step in the electron transport chain. Coenzyme Q (ubiquinone) is an electron carrier which transfers electrons from the NADH dehydroge-nase complex to cytochrome bc1.

## 28. B (Chromatid adhesion and segregation)

The centromere is a region of specialised DNA that is responsible for holding two sister chromatids together. They provide an attachment point for kinetochore fibres to bind and then engage with spindles. This, in turn, provides a point of attachment from which the sister chromatids can be separated by the spindle microtubules during anaphase.

The centrosome is responsible for producing the microtubule organising centre from which spindle microtubules will radiate. Cyclin-dependent kinases can phosphorylate nuclear lamins and stimulate the dissolution of the nuclear envelope. Histone proteins bind to DNA sequences and pro-mote the coiling and condensation of DNA. Cytokinesis occurs during telophase. As a nuclear envelope forms around the two aggregates of chromosomes that are present at the end of anaphase, a cleavage furrow will form at the equator of the cell. This will deepen and, eventually, the cytoplasm of the daughter cells will separate.

## 29.  B (129)

As a 16-carbon compound, palmitic acid has the capacity to yield eight molecules of the 2-carbon compound acetyl-CoA. Therefore, palmitic acid undergoes seven subsequent cycles of beta oxidation in order to generate the maximum available number of acetyl-CoA.

- Palmitic acid (16) is consecutively decarboxylated by the removal of 2 carbon atoms from acyl-CoA resulting in the formation of acetyl-CoA, and a shortened acyl-CoA — 14 carbon atoms long.
- This is repeated for following cycles of beta oxidation until the final 4 carbon acyl-CoA compound is broken into two individual acetyl-CoA molecules.
- Each cycle of beta oxidation yields a single molecule of reduced NAD and FAD, entering into the electron transport chain to produce ATP through oxidative phosphorylation, in addition to the ATP generated directly through the subsequent oxidation of acetyl-CoA.
- Acetyl-CoA can be oxidised in the Krebs cycle provided that beta oxidation and carbohydrate metabolism is balanced (since oxaloacetate is required as a substrate).

$$C_{15}H_{31}COOH+8CoASH+ATP+7FAD^++7NAD^++7H_2O \rightarrow 8CH_3COSCoA+AMP+PPi+7FADH_2+7NADH+7H^+$$

In the example of palmitic acid, each acetyl-CoA yields 12 ATP molecules ($12 \times 8 = 96$), each reduced FAD yields 2 ATP molecules ($2 \times 7 = 14$), each reduced NAD yields 3 ATP molecules ($3 \times 7 = 21$), giving a total of 131 ATP molecules. The process expends 2 ATP molecules, so the net total number of ATP molecules generated is 129.

## 30.  D (Succinate)

The fluid matrix of the mitochondrion contains the enzymes that are responsible for the Krebs cycle. The main function of the Krebs cycle is to use acetyl-CoA to generate ATP. It involves a series of decarboxylation and dehydrogenation reactions. To begin with, acetyl-CoA entering the Krebs cycle will transfer the 2-carbon acetate group to a 4-carbon compound (oxaloacetate), thereby forming citrate (6-carbon). The citrate will then be decarboxylated to α-ketoglutarate, releasing a molecule of carbon dioxide and generating NADH. α-ketoglutarate will also release a carbon dioxide molecule thereby generating 4-carbon succinyl-CoA. Succinyl-CoA is then converted to succinate which generates a molecule of ATP. Succinate is then converted to fumarate which, in turn, is converted to malate and, ultimately, oxaloacetate. A single cycle will, therefore, generate 2 molecules of carbon dioxide, 1 molecule of ATP along with 3 molecules of reduced NAD and 1 molecule of reduced FADH.

# Haematology

## Questions

1. A 43-year-old woman requires a blood transfusion after a laparoscopic cholecystectomy. Her group and screen reveal the presence of IgM Anti-A and IgG Anti-D antibodies.
   Which of the following blood types should be given to this patient?

   A  A+
   B  A–
   C  B+
   D  B–
   E  O–

2. Which of the following is most appropriate to administer in a patient with a low fibrinogen level?

   A  Fresh frozen plasma
   B  Cryoprecipitate
   C  Platelet concentrates
   D  Plasmapheresis
   E  Packed red blood cells

3. A high number of which leukocyte is associated with severe asthma?

   A  Plasma cells
   B  Neutrophils
   C  Eosinophils
   D  Macrophages
   E  CD4⁺ Lymphocytes

4. A 33-year-old man with a background of sickle cell disease has presented to A&E with sudden-onset right-sided chest pain and breathlessness. He had been recovering from a chest infection at home when the pain began. His observations are shown below.

   RR: 24 breaths/min
   $SpO_2$: 92% on air
   HR: 102 bpm
   BP: 128/86 mm Hg
   Temp: 36.4°C

   Which of the following best describes the pathophysiology of his current presentation?

   A  Increased blood flow due to infection resulted in a pulmonary embolism
   B  Reduced oxygenation due to infection resulting in haemoglobin polymerisation and sickling
   C  Overhydration resulting in sickling
   D  Resulting from increased red cell breakdown causing severe anaemia
   E  Local lung damage due to infection has caused pain and breathlessness

5. A 47-year-old man is referred to the outpatient clinic to further investigate his jaundice. He has been investigated for biliary obstruction; however, no cause was identified. He has a background of ischaemic heart disease for which he takes aspirin 75 mg OD. A full blood count is requested ahead of his appointment.

Hb: 83 g/L (135–175)
MCV: 110 fL (82–100)
Reticulocytes: 440 × 10⁹/L (50–100)
Blood film: Macrocytic anaemia with the presence of Heinz bodies
DAT: Negative

What is the most likely cause of his anaemia?

**A** Hereditary spherocytosis
**B** Glucose-6-phosphate dehydrogenase deficiency
**C** Anaemia of chronic disease
**D** Autoimmune haemolytic anaemia
**E** Iron deficiency anaemia

6. A 23-year-old woman is being investigated for a cause of her heavy menstrual bleeding. This has been an issue since her periods began at the age of 13 years. She also has frequent nosebleeds that take a considerable amount of time to stop bleeding. A coagulation screen reveals a normal prothrombin time and a slightly prolonged APTT. Her full blood count reveals a mild microcytic anaemia with no other abnormalities.
   Given the clinical information, what is the most likely diagnosis?

   **A** Idiopathic thrombocytopenic purpura
   **B** Bernard soulier syndrome
   **C** Haemophilia A
   **D** Von Willebrand disease
   **E** Storage pool disease

7. A student has identified a white blood cell during a laboratory practical. It has a bilobed nucleus and prominent cytoplasmic granules.
   Which other feature of the cell would make it more likely to be a basophil than another type of white cell?

   **A** The cell cytoplasm appears to have a blue stain
   **B** The cell is larger than the erythrocytes

    **C**  The cell nucleus is hypersegmented
    **D**  The nucleus is more 'indented' than it is lobed
    **E**  The nucleus occupies the majority of the cell

8.  Which of these has no potential to develop into a white blood cell?

    **A**  Haemocytoblast
    **B**  Common myeloid progenitor
    **C**  Common lymphoid progenitor
    **D**  Megakaryocyte
    **E**  Progranulocyte

9.  Which of the following is low in hereditary haemochromatosis?

    **A**  Iron
    **B**  Hepcidin
    **C**  Transferrin saturation
    **D**  Ferroportin
    **E**  Ferritin

10.  A 72-year-old patient presents to his GP with a long history of tiredness. A blood test is requested revealing the following results.

Hb: 96 g/L (135–175)
MCV: 86 fL (82–100)
WBC: $21.3 \times 10^9$/L (4–11)
Neut: $17.1 \times 10^9$/L (2–7)
Lymph: $2.4 \times 10^9$/L (1.5–4)

Chromosomal analysis reveals the presence of the BCR-ABL1 gene, and the patient goes on to be treated with a tyrosine kinase inhibitor. What is the most likely diagnosis?

    **A**  Acute lymphoblastic leukaemia
    **B**  Acute myeloid leukaemia

**C** Chronic lymphocytic leukaemia
**D** Chronic myeloid leukaemia
**E** Multiple myeloma

11. A 19-year-old girl visits her GP after feeling generally unwell with a sore throat for the preceding 2 weeks. A blood test is conducted which reveals a raised lymphocyte count and her blood film report mentions the presence of atypical lymphocytes with basophilic cytoplasm and scalloped margins.
What is the most likely diagnosis?

    **A** Folic acid deficiency
    **B** Chronic lymphocytic leukaemia
    **C** Epstein–Barr virus
    **D** Sideroblastic anaemia
    **E** HIV infection

12. A 42-year-old man has just undergone an open valve replacement for a damaged aortic valve. A mechanical valve was inserted, and the patient has been told that he will have to be on warfarin for the rest of his life.
Which of the following is true regarding his warfarin treatment?

    **A** The dose of warfarin should be fixed indefinitely
    **B** Low molecular weight heparin should be co-prescribed at the start of treatment
    **C** Recommend a diet that is rich in vitamin K
    **D** The anticoagulant effect of warfarin is most potent within two days of commencing treatment
    **E** Warfarin does not require regular monitoring

13. A 55-year-old patient has undergone a gastrectomy due to stomach cancer. A blood film is taken.
Which of the following types of anaemia is most likely to be seen in this patient?

     **A** Microcytic anaemia
     **B** Megaloblastic anaemia
     **C** Normocytic anaemia
     **D** Anaemia of chronic disease
     **E** Aplastic anaemia

14. Which of the following treatments for Von Willebrand disease will cause an increase in circulating Von Willebrand factor levels?

     **A** Tranexamic acid
     **B** Prednisolone
     **C** Desmopressin
     **D** Apixaban
     **E** Factor VIII concentrate

15. Which of the following statements are true regarding red blood cell destruction?

     **A** Phagocytic macrophages within the liver consume the erythrocytes
     **B** The normal lifespan of a red cell is 180 days
     **C** Globin is metabolised to carbohydrates
     **D** Haem is metabolised to bilirubin and $Fe^{2+}$
     **E** Bilirubin is excreted exclusively in the faeces

16. The blood film of a patient attending the haematology clinic is being analysed in the laboratory. The key finding is the presence of Auer rods within abnormal cells.
    Given the most likely diagnosis, which of the following statements is true?

     **A** Caused by a mutation in a gene encoding a signalling protein
     **B** Cell kinetics and function are not significantly affected
     **C** There is an increased production of end-lineage cells
     **D** Robertsonian translocation between chromosomes 9 and 22
     **E** Associated with neutropenia

17. A 56-year-old woman has been admitted to the acute medical unit with pyrexia of unknown origin. A septic screen has revealed no obvious locus of infection and the patient remains unwell despite treatment with broad-spectrum antibiotics. She has developed widespread ecchymoses across her limbs. She has been previously well with no past medical history and no regular medications. A coagulation screen reveals the following results.

    PT: 38 seconds (9.6–11.6)
    APTT: 54 seconds (26–32)

    Given the clinical information, what is the most likely cause of these symptoms?

    **A** Disseminated intravascular coagulation
    **B** Haemophilia A
    **C** Haemophilia B
    **D** Von Willebrand disease
    **E** Idiopathic thrombocytopaenic purpura

18. A third-year medical student takes blood from a patient and runs the sample to the laboratory for a full blood count. The initial result revealed that the patient had a haemoglobin of 88 g/L. The blood test was repeated the following day and the patient's haemoglobin had risen to 104 g/L.
    Which of the following could explain this result?

    **A** The patient has polycythaemia vera
    **B** The patient had been receiving IV fluids
    **C** The patient had a massive bleed before the first sample
    **D** The patient has leukaemia
    **E** The patient has peripheral vascular disease

19. A 59-year-old man is admitted to the major trauma unit after being in a car accident. He is on lifelong warfarin after having a mechanical valve replacement several years ago. His INR is 7.3 and he needs rapid reversal of his warfarin. An urgent fresh frozen plasma transfusion is arranged.

Which type of blood plasma should be transfused?

   **A** A+
   **B** AB+
   **C** AB−
   **D** O−
   **E** O+

20. Which factor binds to tissue factor to activate the coagulation cascade?

   **A** XII
   **B** X
   **C** IX
   **D** V
   **E** VII

21. A 33-year-old man is being investigated further after a blood test at his GP practice revealed that he was anaemic. The blood film report stated there was a considerable degree of anisocytosis.
    What is the definition of anisocytosis?

   **A** Variation in red cell colour
   **B** Variation in red cell shape
   **C** Variation in red cell size
   **D** Variation in red cell number
   **E** Variation in red cell aggregation

22. A 54-year-old man visits his GP complaining of an intractable itch. He says that his whole body has been itching all over for the last 6 months and emollients have not brought him any relief. On examination, he has a ruddy complexion and widespread excoriation marks but no visible rash. A full blood count reveals a raised haemoglobin (187 g/L).
    What is the most likely diagnosis?

A  Thalassemia beta
B  Polycythaemia vera
C  Chronic kidney disease
D  Chronic myeloid leukaemia
E  Acute lymphoblastic leukaemia

23. A 26-year-old man has recently returned from a backpacking holiday in the Democratic Republic of Congo. He has had persistent fevers over the past 2 weeks since his return. A thick and thin blood film confirms a diagnosis of falciparum malaria.
Which of the following additional blood test findings are likely to be present?

A  Transient neutropenia
B  Persistent lymphocytosis
C  Transient monocytosis
D  Persistent basophilia
E  Transient eosinophilia

24. What is the mechanism of action of clopidogrel?

A  Irreversibly inhibits cyclooxygenase
B  Enhances the action of antithrombin III
C  Inhibits vitamin K epoxide reductase
D  Irreversibly inhibits the $P2Y_{12}$ receptor
E  Directly inhibits factor Xa

25. A 64-year-old woman visits her GP with complaints of ongoing tiredness. For the last 6 months, she has felt tired throughout the day and is unable to tolerate her normal level of activity. She has also developed a 'pins and needles' sensation in her hands and feet. Her past medical history includes well-controlled hypothyroidism and vitiligo. A blood test reveals the following results.

Hb: 69 g/L (115–155)
MCV: 112 fL (82–100)

WBC: $4.2 \times 10^9$/L (4–11)

Reticulocytes: $60 \times 10^9$/L (50–100)

Blood film: Significant number of megaloblasts with hypersegmented neutrophils and poikilocytosis

What is the most likely cause of her anaemia?

A  Iron deficiency

B  Vitamin B12 deficiency

C  Autoimmune haemolytic anaemia

D  Paroxysmal nocturnal haemoglobinuria

E  Microangiopathic haemolytic anaemia

26. Which of the following statements is correct regarding neutrophils?

    A  They migrate into tissues upon production

    B  They are round

    C  Their main function is signalling

    D  They take 2–3 days to reach the site of injury

    E  They are chemotactic

27. The synthesis of which clotting factors are directly affected by warfarin?

    A  II, V, VII, VIII

    B  II, V, VII, IX

    C  II, VII, VIII, IX

    D  II, VII, IX, X

    E  II, VII, X, XI

28. Which four of the following treatments or blood products are likely to be used in the treatment of acute lymphoblastic leukaemia?

    1. Red cells

    2. Platelets

    3. Antibiotics

**4.** Cryoprecipitate
**5.** Systemic and intrathecal chemotherapy

**A** 1, 2, 3, 4
**B** 2, 3, 4, 5
**C** 1, 3, 4, 5
**D** 1, 2, 4, 5
**E** 1, 2, 3, 5

29. A 77-year-old woman was admitted to the surgical ward after having an episode of severe rectal bleeding. She underwent a colonoscopy which reveals a bleeding arteriovenous malformation which was subsequently cauterised. Her haemoglobin on admission was 64 g/L and it rose to 89 g/L after receiving 2 units of packed red cells. A blood test three days later, prior to discharge, revealed a haemoglobin concentration of 79 g/L. She had not had any further episodes of rectal bleeding during her admission. She had, however, developed an AKI and received 3 L of IV fluids.

    Which of the following red cell parameters would be most useful in determining the likely cause of her drop in haemoglobin?

    **A** Packed cell volume
    **B** Red cell distribution width
    **C** Mean cell volume
    **D** Mean cell haemoglobin
    **E** Mean cell haemoglobin concentration

30. A 54-year-old woman has visited her GP complaining of feeling increasingly tired towards the end of the day. She feels that this has been getting worse over the last 3 weeks. She has also noticed that she becomes more breathless than usual when climbing the stairs in her house. On examination, she is noted to be tachycardic with conjunctival pallor and some mild yellowing of the sclerae. A full blood count reveals the following results.

    Hb: 86 g/L (115–155)
    MCV: 92 fL (82–100)

WBC: $7.1 \times 10^9$/L (4–11)
Neut: $3.1 \times 10^9$/L (2–7)
CRP: 0.6 (<0.6)
Reticulocytes: 10% (0.5–1)

What is the most likely diagnosis?

A  Sickle cell disease
B  Autoimmune haemolytic anaemia
C  Aplastic anaemia
D  Thalassemia
E  Gilbert syndrome

# Answers

## 1. D (B–)

Patients who require a blood transfusion need to have a blood test called a 'Group and Screen' which involves identifying the patient's ABO and Rhesus blood type and checking for the presence of antibodies against red blood cell antigens. People will have naturally occurring antibodies against the A and/or B antigens that they do not possess on their own red cell membranes (i.e. someone who has group A blood, will have naturally existing anti-B antibodies). People who do not have Rhesus D antigens (denoted by the + or – sign) can develop anti-D antibodies following exposure to Rhesus-positive blood. This can happen during pregnancy or following a blood transfusion. Except for in emergencies, patients should have a group and screen and blood of an appropriate type should be issued. O– blood does not have any of the important red cell antigens and, therefore, can be transfused to patients of any blood group. It is, however, in short supply and should only be used in emergencies where there is not enough time to conduct a group and screen or cross match.

## 2. B (Cryoprecipitate)

Cryoprecipitate is a blood product prepared from plasma that contains fibrinogen, Von Willebrand factor, factor VIII, factor XIII and fibronectin. It tends to be used in critically ill patients with low fibrinogen levels, for example, due to disseminated intravascular coagulation.

Fresh frozen plasma contains all the major plasma proteins and tends to be used in patients who are deficient in coagulation factors. It can also be used for the reversal of anticoagulation (e.g. due to warfarin). Platelet concentrates are used when platelet levels are low (e.g. idiopathic thrombocytopaenic purpura). Plasmapheresis is a process by which plasma is passed through a machine which filters out abnormal proteins (e.g. antibodies in myasthenia gravis) before returning the filtered plasma to the body. Packed red cells are used in patients who have lost a significant amount of blood and in patients who are profoundly anaemic.

### 3. C (Eosinophils)

Asthma is an atopic condition and, if triggered by an allergen, is considered a type I hypersensitivity reaction. The presentation of an allergen by antigen-presenting cells to Th0 cells leads to T-helper cell differentiation. This eventually results in the secretion of IL5 which promotes maturation and the release of eosinophils.

Plasma cells are important in the production of target-specific antibodies. Neutrophils are the first responders to infection or injury. The presence of an abundance of neutrophils is the hallmark of acute inflammation. Macrophages are derived from monocytes and are the predominant phagocytic cells that engulf pathogens. CD4+ cells are an important component of the acquired immune response. They recognise peptides presented on MHC Class II molecules on antigen-presenting cells.

### 4. B (Reduced oxygenation due to infection resulting in haemoglobin polymerisation and sickling)

Sickle cell disease is an autosomal recessive condition that is caused by a single gene mutation that results in the exchange of glutamate for valine in the beta-globin gene. This results in the production of haemoglobin S which is prone to polymerisation under precipitating conditions such as dehydration and hypoxia. HbS polymerisation leads to sickling of the cell which, in turn, increases the risk of blood vessel occlusion. The sudden-onset chest pain and breathlessness in the context of a chest infection is suggestive of acute chest syndrome. This is a complication of sickle cell disease which is caused by vaso-occlusion within the pulmonary vasculature. The chest infection can cause local tissue hypoxia which results in sickling.

Increased blood flow would not increase the risk of pulmonary embolism. Dehydration can precipitate sickling. Patients with sickle cell disease are usually anaemic due to increased red cell turnover, however, this would cause chronic breathlessness and reduced exercise tolerance. Local lung damage due to infection can cause breathlessness but it would not cause sudden-onset chest pain.

## 5. B (Glucose-6-phosphate dehydrogenase deficiency)

Glucose-6-phosphate dehydrogenase (G6PD) deficiency is a form of haemolytic anaemia that results from an inability of red cells to generate glutathione. Glutathione is the red cell's main defence mechanism against oxidative damage, so a deficiency of glutathione results in increased susceptibility to oxidative damage and cell death. Heinz bodies are lumps of denatured haemoglobin within red cells — they are a marker of oxidative damage. Haemolysis can be precipitated by various agents that can increase the risk of oxidative damage (e.g. antimalarial drugs). An increase in red cell breakdown means that there will be an increase in bilirubin generation. This will exceed the capacity of the liver to metabolise bilirubin, so it will manifest as jaundice.

Hereditary spherocytosis is an inherited disorder of the red cell membrane which results in spherical red blood cells that have lost their biconcave shape. Spherocytes can be identified on a blood film. Anaemia of chronic disease is a disease entity in which anaemia occurs on a background of chronic disease (e.g. rheumatoid arthritis). It is thought to occur due to the abundance of proinflammatory cytokines (e.g. IL-1 and TNF-$\alpha$) in chronic disease. These cytokines suppress the absorption and transport of iron, thereby limiting the ability of the body to use this iron in red cell production. Autoimmune haemolytic anaemia is a disorder in which red cells are broken down by autoantibodies. A direct antiglobulin test (DAT) can detect the presence of antibodies directed against red cell antigens. Iron deficiency anaemia would cause microcytic anaemia. It would not cause jaundice as it is caused by insufficient production of red cells as opposed to excessive breakdown.

## 6. D (Von Willebrand disease)

Von Willebrand Disease is characterised by the reduced or abnormal production of Von Willebrand Factor (VWF). VWF is important in facilitating platelet adhesion to a site of injury and it stabilises factor VIII, thereby preventing premature degradation. There are three main types of Von Willebrand Disease: Type 1 — reduced VWF, Type 2 — defective VWF,

Type 3 — total absence of VWF. It typically manifests as easy bruising, frequent and prolonged nosebleeds, prolonged bleeding from cuts, heavy periods and excessive bleeding after surgery.

Idiopathic thrombocytopenic purpura is caused by the generation of anti-bodies directed at platelets. It results in easy bruising due to thrombocy-topaenia that may manifest as petechiae. Bernard-Soulier syndrome is a rare inherited clotting disorder characterised by unusually large platelets, thrombocytopaenia and prolonged bleeding time. It is caused by a defi-ciency in glycoprotein Ib, which is responsible for enabling the binding of platelets to VWF. Haemophilia A is an X-linked recessive disorder char-acterised by factor VIII deficiency. This results in a prolonged APTT and a propensity for deep bleeding (e.g. haemarthrosis). Storage pool disease is caused by an absence of ADP-containing dense granules within plate-lets. This results in impaired platelet activation and aggregation.

### 7.  A (The cell cytoplasm appears to have a blue stain)

Basophils are a type of white cell which has a characteristic bi-lobed nucleus and dense cytoplasmic granules that stain blue. They are impor-tant in allergic reactions and parasitic infections. All leukocytes, other than lymphocytes, are larger than erythrocytes, which are ~7 micrometres in diameter.

A hypersegmented nucleus may be found in a neutrophil. They are associ-ated with megaloblastic anaemia as a result of vitamin B12 or folic acid deficiency. An indented nucleus is a feature of a monocyte. The nucleus would occupy the majority of the cell in lymphocytes.

### 8.  D (Megakaryocyte)

A megakaryocyte is a large cell, found in the bone marrow, that gives rise to platelets.

Haemocytoblasts or multipotential hematopoietic stem cells have the capacity to develop into any type of blood cell. Common myeloid progenitor cells are cellular precursors for mast cells and myeloblasts (the latter is a precursor for granulocytes and monocytes). Common lymphoid progenitor cells are cellular precursors for natural killer cells and all lymphocytes — B-cells, T-cells and plasma cells. Progranulocytes have the capacity to differentiate into basophils, neutrophils and eosinophils.

## 9. B (Hepcidin)

Hereditary haemochromatosis is a condition in which patients become iron overloaded. This can result in damage to a number of organs manifesting in conditions such as cirrhosis, diabetes mellitus and heart failure. In hereditary haemochromatosis, the C282Y mutation leads to inappropriately low hepcidin expression. Hepcidin is a regulatory protein that can reduce iron absorption within the gastrointestinal tract. Usually when serum iron levels are high, hepcidin levels will be high, thereby reducing intestinal iron absorption. Inadequate levels of hepcidin, however, will render this mechanism ineffective, resulting in excessive absorption of iron. This gives rise to a high serum iron, high ferritin and high transferrin saturation.

## 10. D (Chronic myeloid leukaemia)

Chronic myeloid leukaemia (CML) is a haematological malignancy affecting the myeloid lineage of white cells. It results from a Robertsonian translocation between chromosomes 9 and 22, resulting in the formation of the BCR-ABL1 gene. This leads to excessive tyrosine kinase activity and expansion of this lineage of cells. It may be asymptomatic; however, it can also present with features of bone marrow failure (anaemia, bruising due to thrombocytopaenia and recurrent infections due to reduced numbers of functional leukocytes). CML can undergo a blast transformation by which it turns into an acute myeloid leukaemia. Tyrosine kinase inhibitors (e.g. imatinib) are the treatment of choice for CML.

Acute lymphoblastic leukaemia is the most common malignancy in childhood. It presents relatively acutely with features of bone marrow failure. The peripheral blood film will reveal the presence of large numbers of lymphoblasts. Acute myeloid leukaemia is more common in adults and will also present with features of bone marrow failure. The blood film will reveal a large number of myeloblasts. Like CML, chronic lymphocytic leukaemia may also present insidiously with features of bone marrow failure. It is characterised by a clonal expansion of mature lymphocytes. Multiple myeloma is a malignancy of plasma cells. The symptoms it causes tend to be related to the presence of massive amounts of a single type of immunoglobulin. It can cause lytic bone lesions and pathological fractures, hypercalcaemia, renal failure, anaemia and hypercoagulability.

### 11.  C (Epstein–Barr virus)

Lymphocytosis is a feature of any viral infection. Epstein–Barr virus is a common virus that causes glandular fever (also known as infectious mononucleosis). It is particularly common in teenagers and young adults. The classical features include a fever, sore throat and tiredness. A blood film would reveal atypical lymphocytes — these are large with basophilic cytoplasm and scalloped margins. The membrane may appear to hug nearby erythrocytes. Folic acid deficiency can cause megaloblastic anaemia. This is associated with the presence of megaloblasts (large, immature red blood cells) and hypersegmented nuclei.

Chronic lymphocytic leukaemia results in very high numbers of a single lineage of mature white cells. It typically occurs in older patients and may be asymptomatic. Sideroblastic anaemia is a cause of microcytic anaemia that results from an inability of red cells to incorporate iron into haemoglobin. It is characterised by the presence of rings around the nucleus. HIV would cause a low lymphocyte (CD4) count.

### 12.  B (Low molecular weight heparin should be co-prescribed at the start of treatment)

Warfarin is an anticoagulant that has been used in the treatment or prevention of various diseases. Direct oral anticoagulants (e.g. apixaban) are beginning to supersede warfarin in a number of settings, however, several patients do continue to use warfarin. It is a vitamin K epoxide reductase inhibitor which prevents the gamma-carboxylation of clotting factors II, VII, IX and X. It is an oral medication that requires regular INR monitoring to ensure that its anticoagulant effect remains within the therapeutic window. In addition to the aforementioned clotting factors, warfarin also inhibits protein C and protein S, which are part of the body's endogenous anticoagulant mechanism. This means that warfarin actually induces a prothrombotic state for the first few days after commencing treatment. For this reason, low molecular weight heparin (e.g. tinzaparin) may be co-prescribed until the INR is found to be stable within the therapeutic range.

Warfarin requires regular INR monitoring and the dose may be adjusted depending on the INR. Vitamin K is used to reverse the effects of warfarin. Warfarin has a pro-coagulant effect within the first few days of commencing treatment.

### 13. B (Megaloblastic anaemia)

A gastrectomy is a surgical procedure in which part or all of the stomach is removed. It may be performed due to stomach cancer or morbid obesity. Once ingested, vitamin B12 will bind to intrinsic factor (a transport protein released by gastric parietal cells). Intrinsic factor prevents B12 degradation and transports it to the terminal ileum where it is absorbed. Following absorption, it will bind to transcobalamin II which transports B12 via the blood to the liver or to other tissues. A patient who has had a gastrectomy will be unable to produce intrinsic factor, thereby resulting in B12 deficiency. B12 is essential for DNA synthesis, so a deficiency results in impaired nuclear maturation and cell division within the bone marrow. This results in the release of large, immature red blood cells in the circulation, known as megaloblasts.

Causes of microcytic anaemia include iron deficiency, thalassemia, anaemia of chronic disease and sideroblastic anaemia. Causes of normocytic anaemia include an acute bleed, splenic sequestration and aplastic anaemia. Anaemia of chronic disease refers to the development of anaemia on a background of chronic disease. It is thought to arise due to a negative effect exerted by proinflammatory cytokines on iron utilisation. Aplastic anaemia is a disease in which bone marrow output suddenly stops. This may be seen in the context of parvovirus B19 infection in patients with sickle cell disease. The sudden reduction in blood cell output results in a normocytic anaemia.

### 14.  C (Desmopressin)

Von Willebrand Disease type 1 and 3 are caused by a partial or complete deficiency of Von Willebrand Factor (VWF). VWF adheres to exposed collagen fibres under damaged endothelium and mediates the binding of platelets via the glycoprotein Ib receptor. Desmopressin is a vasopressin analogue that is commonly used in the treatment of cranial diabetes insipidus. It has also been noted to stimulate the release of VWF from endothelial cells, so it may be used in the treatment of Von Willebrand Disease. This can also bring about an increase in factor VIII levels as VWF is responsible for stabilising factor VIII.

Tranexamic acid is an antifibrinolytic that prevents the activation of plasmin and improves clot maintenance. It is often used in bleeding trauma patients. Prednisolone is a steroid that can be used in the treatment of immune thrombocytopaenic purpura as it can suppress antibody production. Apixaban is a direct oral anticoagulant (DOAC) that works by inhibiting factor Xa. It is often used in the treatment of atrial fibrillation and venous thromboembolism. Factor VIII concentrate may be used in treating Von Willebrand Disease Type 3; however, it would not cause an increase in VWF.

### 15.  D (Haem is metabolised to bilirubin and $Fe^{2+}$)

Red blood cells last around 120 days within the circulation, after which they are destroyed by phagocytic cells in the spleen. The haem is removed and biliverdin is released. This will eventually be converted into bilirubin. Iron ($Fe^{2+}$) will also be released which will get transported to the bone marrow to be used in the synthesis of new red cells or it may be stored by ferritin.

Globin is hydrolysed into amino acids, which are returned to the bone marrow for erythropoiesis. Bilirubin is transported to the liver where it will be conjugated with glucuronide to create water-soluble, conjugated bilirubin. This is then excreted into the duodenum. The conjugated bilirubin is acted upon by colonic bacteria to produce urobilinogen and stercobilinogen. This is excreted in the faeces, however, some urobilinogen is reabsorbed within the gastrointestinal tract and excreted by the kidneys.

## 16. E (Associated with neutropenia)

Auer rods are a classical finding in acute myeloid leukaemia. They are needle-shaped bodies that are found within the cytoplasm of myeloblasts or progranulocytes as a result of abnormal fusion of primary granules. Although acute myeloid leukaemia causes excessive release of myeloblasts from the bone marrow, it results in a decrease in the total number of functional neutrophils. This is because the predominance of one clone of myeloblasts impairs the ability of the bone marrow to produce other, functional blood cells. It will also cause thrombocytopaenia and anaemia.

## 17. A (Disseminated intravascular coagulation)

Disseminated intravascular coagulation (DIC) is a condition in which widespread activation of the clotting cascade results in the formation of blood clots across the body associated with the rapid consumption of clotting factors. Although this may seem to be a prothrombotic state, the consumption of clotting factors results in severe hypocoagulability. It can be triggered by a number of stimuli including malignancy, infection and pregnancy. On a coagulation screen, it is likely to cause a significant prolongation of PT and APTT.

Haemophilia A and B are X-linked disorders (hence, very unlikely to present in a woman) in which patients are unable to produce factor 8 or 9 respectively. It would cause a prolonged APTT and is likely to present earlier in life with complications related to excessive or abnormal bleeding. Von Willebrand disease is an inherited condition characterised by reduced or abnormal Von Willebrand factor (VWF) production. VWF is a protein that is responsible for helping platelets to bind to sites of endothelial injury. Furthermore, it is important for the stability of factor VIII. Investigations may reveal a low factor VIII level and prolonged APTT. Idiopathic thrombocytopenic purpura (ITP) is characterised by the presence of antibodies directed against platelets. This results in enhanced phagocytosis of platelets by macrophages.

## 18.  B (The patient had been receiving IV fluids)

Giving patients large volumes of fluids can result in a dilutional anaemia. This is because the same number of red cells and, hence, same amount of haemoglobin, is diluted in a larger pool of fluid. It is also important to ensure that blood is not taken from an arm that is being used to administer fluids, as this can lead to spurious urea and electrolyte results.

Polycythaemia vera is a condition in which patients have high haemoglobin levels due to excessive proliferation of red cells. If a patient has a massive bleed, it is unlikely to show a change in haemoglobin until sufficient time has elapsed for the patient's body to retain enough fluid to replenish their circulating volume. Both plasma and red cells are lost in a massive bleed so the concentration of haemoglobin may remain the same initially. Patients with leukaemia are often anaemic as their bone marrow is unable to produce a sufficient output of red cells, however, this is unlikely to correct itself overnight. Peripheral vascular disease would not affect haemoglobin.

## 19.  B (AB+)

Plasma is the component of blood that contains the serum and plasma proteins. It will, therefore, contain any pre-existing antibodies against red blood cell antigens. AB+ plasma is considered the universal plasma donor as a donor who has AB+ blood will have no antibodies against A, B or Rhesus D. If rapid reversal of warfarin is required in an emergency situation and there is insufficient time to conduct a full group and screen, AB+ plasma may be used.

## 20. E (VII)

Tissue factor is the trigger for the extrinsic pathway of clotting cascade activation. After being released from a damaged endothelium, tissue factor will bind to factor VII, thereby activating it to factor VIIa. Activated factor VII will then catalyse the activation of factor X to Xa.

## 21. C (Variation in red cell size)

Anisocytosis is defined as a variation in red cell size. In a healthy individual, all red cells should be the same size. Anisocytosis can occur in the context of micro- and macrocytosis. Anisocytosis with microcytosis may be due to iron deficiency. Anisocytosis with macrocytosis may be due to vitamin B12 or folate deficiency. Poikilocytosis refers to variation in red cell shape. This can arise due to a number of causes including iron deficiency anaemia, alcoholism and chronic liver disease.

## 22. B (Polycythaemia vera)

Polycythaemia vera is a rare myeloproliferative condition characterised by an overproduction of red blood cells. It is caused by an activating mutation of a tyrosine kinase gene (JAK2). Polycythaemia vera often manifests with itching and thrombosis (due to hypercoagulability). A full blood count is likely to reveal a high haemoglobin with a high haematocrit. Definitive diagnosis is established by testing for the JAK2 mutation.

Thalassemia beta is an inherited disorder of globin production that causes microcytic anaemia. Chronic kidney disease can lead to anaemia as the diseased kidneys are less able to produce erythropoietin. Chronic myeloid leukaemia is likely to cause anaemia as the expansion of the malignant clone of myeloid cells can crowd out other haematopoietic cells from the bone marrow, resulting in bone marrow failure. Acute lymphoblastic leukaemia is characterised by an abnormal proliferation of lymphoblasts. It, too, will crowd out other haematopoietic cells from the bone marrow thereby resulting in bone marrow failure.

### 23. E (Transient eosinophilia)

Eosinophils are a subset of white cells that are involved in allergy and immune responses to parasites (e.g. malaria). A parasitic infection would, therefore, cause a transient eosinophilia.

Neutrophils are the primary acute inflammatory cells that are first recruited in any infectious or inflammatory condition. Neutrophils are mainly involved in tackling bacterial infections; however, the neutrophil count is likely to be raised in malaria. Malaria typically causes lymphopenia. Monocytosis is usually associated with chronic bacterial infections. Persistent basophilia is associated with chronic myeloid leukaemia.

### 24. D (Irreversibly inhibits the $P2Y_{12}$ receptor)

Clopidogrel is an antiplatelet that is commonly used in the treatment of ischaemic heart disease. It is a selective inhibitor of the $P2Y_{12}$ receptor. It prevents the binding of ADP, thereby inhibiting a conformational change in the platelet. This, in turn, results in impaired glycoprotein IIb/IIIa expression and, hence, platelet aggregation.

Aspirin is another commonly used antiplatelet that irreversibly inhibits the cyclooxygenase (COX) enzyme and, therefore, inhibits the production of the prothrombotic factor, thromboxane A2. Heparin is an anticoagulant that works by binding to antithrombin III and potentiating its action. Antithrombin III is part of the body's endogenous anticoagulant mechanism. It inactivates several clotting factors including factors II, IX, X and XI. Warfarin is an anticoagulant that inhibits vitamin K epoxide reductase, thereby preventing the gamma-carboxylation of factors II, VII, IX and X. Direct oral anticoagulants (e.g. apixaban) work by directly inhibiting certain clotting factors (usually factor Xa).

### 25. B (Vitamin B12 deficiency)

Megaloblasts are large, immature red cells that are associated with anaemia caused by vitamin B12 and folate deficiency. B12 is an essential component of DNA synthesis so deficiency results in impaired nuclear maturation and cell division within the bone marrow. Although the patient is anaemic, their reticulocyte count would be low or normal as they do not have sufficient supplies to be able to produce reticulocytes. B12 deficiency may be due to insufficient dietary intake or due to an inability to absorb B12. Pernicious anaemia is a disease in which a lack of intrinsic factor production by gastric parietal cells results in low B12 levels. It is an autoimmune condition which should be considered in anaemic patients with a background of other autoimmune diseases (e.g. hypothyroidism, vitiligo). B12 is also necessary for myelin formation within the nervous system. Deficiency can, therefore, result in neurological symptoms such as peripheral neuropathy and paraesthesia.

Iron deficiency would cause microcytic anaemia. Autoimmune haemolytic anaemia is caused by the generation of antibodies that target red cell antigens. It may be idiopathic, but it may also occur in the context of lymphoproliferative and autoimmune diseases. It would cause a raised reticulocyte count as the body attempts to compensate for increased red cell breakdown by increasing its output of red blood cells, even if they are immature. A direct antiglobulin test (DAT) can identify these antibodies. Paroxysmal nocturnal haemoglobinuria is a rare condition characterised by haemolytic anaemia, red discolouration of the urine, thrombosis and impaired bone marrow function. Microangiopathic haemolytic anaemia is a form of haemolytic anaemia in which red blood cells lyse due to the shear forces encountered as they pass through small blood vessels. It would cause a raised reticulocyte count.

## 26. E (They are chemotactic)

Neutrophils are lobulated cells that remain active within circulation for up to 10 hours before migrating into tissues via chemotaxis. They are the first immune cells to reach the site of injury whereby it phagocytoses pathogens and releases various chemotactic mediators that promote further inflammatory cell recruitment.

## 27. D (II, VII, IX, X)

Warfarin is a commonly used anticoagulant that acts by inhibiting vitamin K epoxide reductase. This prevents the gamma-carboxylation of factors II,

VII, IX and X, which is required for these clotting factors to be fully functional. Warfarin also inhibits protein C and protein S which are part of the body's endogenous anticoagulant mechanism. This means that, within the first few days of commencing warfarin treatment, the patient will actually be in a hypercoagulable state. Low molecular weight heparin is usually co-prescribed during these first few days to mitigate this effect.

## 28. E (1, 2, 3, 5)

Acute lymphoblastic leukaemia (ALL) is a haematological malignancy characterised by excessive production of a clone of lymphoblasts within the bone marrow. This results in the appearance of lymphoblasts in peripheral blood and the crowding out of other haematopoietic cells from the bone marrow — thereby resulting in bone marrow failure (anaemia, thrombocytopaenia and recurrent infections). Anaemia can be treated with blood transfusions, thrombocytopaenia with platelet transfusions and recurrent infections with antibiotics. Systemic or intrathecal chemotherapy is likely to be used to treat the disease itself. Cryoprecipitate is a blood product that contains fibrinogen, factor VIII, XIII and Von Willebrand Factor. It is used in various conditions that are characterised by low fibrinogen levels, such as disseminated intravascular coagulation.

## 29. A (Packed cell volume)

Patients who have received large volumes of fluid can develop a dilutional anaemia. This occurs because the same number of haemoglobin/red cells has been diluted in a relatively larger volume of fluid. Packed cell volume (also known as haematocrit) is a measure of the percentage of whole blood that is composed of cells. A decrease in packed cell volume would be suggestive of an increase in the plasma component of the blood (in this case due to the administration of large volumes of IV fluids).

## 30. B (Autoimmune haemolytic anaemia)

This patient has presented with signs and symptoms of anaemia (shortness of breath, reduced exercise tolerance, fatigue, tachycardia and conjunctival pallor). The most important discriminator in this question is the raised reticulocyte count. Reticulocytes are immature red cells which are released prematurely from the bone marrow in response to an increased demand. This typically occurs in the context of a sudden increase in red cell breakdown such as haemolytic anaemia. In this case, a sickle cell splenic sequestration crisis or autoimmune haemolytic anaemia could cause an acute anaemia with a reticulocyte response. Autoimmune haemolytic anaemia is caused by the generation of autoantibodies against red cell antigens. It may be idiopathic, or it may occur secondary to various other haematological conditions such as chronic lymphocytic leukaemia.

A splenic sequestration crisis in sickle cell disease could cause this clinical picture, however, it is very unlikely for a patient to present with sickle cell disease for the first time at the age of 54 years. Aplastic anaemia is a condition in which the bone marrow is unable to produce any cells. This can also occur in the context of sickle cell disease due to parvovirus B19 infection. The virus can inhibit blood cell production in the bone marrow for a relatively short period of time — this does not usually cause problems in healthy individuals, however, the red cells of people with sickle cell disease have a much shorter life span (~20 days) so it can result in an aplastic crisis during which they become profoundly anaemic. The reticulocyte count would be low in aplastic anaemia. Thalassemia is an inherited condition in which the genes for globin production are mutated. It would result in a reduced output of red cells and a low reticulocyte count. Gilbert syndrome is a benign inherited condition caused by an impairment in the ability of the liver to conjugate bilirubin. It does not cause anaemia.

# Immunology and Microbiology

## Questions

1. A newborn baby is noted to be jaundiced soon after birth. The notes from antenatal screening state that the mother is Rhesus D negative and did not receive anti-D immunoglobulin as she failed to attend her scheduled appointments. This is her second child. Her first pregnancy was uneventful.

   Which of the following types of immune response is occurring in this scenario?

   A Type I hypersensitivity
   B Type II hypersensitivity
   C Type III hypersensitivity
   D Type IV hypersensitivity
   E Type V hypersensitivity

2. Which of the following cells is classically associated with acute inflammation?

   A Macrophage
   B Eosinophil
   C Neutrophil

    **D** Mast cell
    **E** CD8+ T-cell

3. Immune dysregulation polyendocrinopathy enteropathy X-linked (IPEX) syndrome is an autoimmune disorder characterised by a Foxp3 mutation.
   Which immune cell is deficient in IPEX syndrome?

    **A** T-helper I cell
    **B** T-helper II cell
    **C** CD8+ T-cell
    **D** T-regulatory cell
    **E** Natural killer cell

4. A 68-year-old woman is admitted to the general medical ward with new-onset confusion and a dry cough. Her chest X-ray shows irregular patchy consolidation in keeping with atypical pneumonia. Urinary antigen testing confirms a diagnosis of *Legionella* pneumonia.
   Which of the following classes of antibiotics is most appropriate in the treatment of atypical pneumonia?

    **A** Aminoglycosides
    **B** Fluoroquinolones
    **C** Macrolides
    **D** Cephalosporins
    **E** Glycopeptides

5. VDJ recombination is a process that determines the specificity of T-cell and B-cell receptors.
   In which lymphoid organ does this process take place for B-cells?

    **A** Thymus gland
    **B** Bone marrow
    **C** Spleen
    **D** Peyer's patches
    **E** Lymph nodes

6. A 51-year-old man with a chronic cough has recently had a chest X-ray which revealed an abnormal nodule in the periphery of his lung. A biopsy was taken which revealed a granuloma.
   Which of the following is most closely associated with this type of pathology?

   **A** Vasodilation and increased vascular permeability
   **B** Histamine release
   **C** Complete resolution
   **D** Mononuclear cell infiltrate
   **E** Neutrophil recruitment

7. Which costimulatory factor is highly expressed by cancer cells to downregulate the immune response?

   **A** PDL-I
   **B** B7
   **C** FASL
   **D** AIRE
   **E** P53

8. A 32-year-old woman has been admitted to the intensive care unit with severe sepsis of unknown origin. A blood culture grows *Staphylococcus aureus*.
   Which of the following proteins allows *Staphylococcus aureus* to evade antibody-mediated phagocytosis?

   **A** Staphylococcal complement inhibitor
   **B** Protein A
   **C** Factor H
   **D** Chemotaxis inhibitory protein
   **E** Staphylococcal superantigen-like protein 7

9. A 33-year-old woman has presented to her GP with a 6-month history of tiredness, depression and irregular periods. Her thyroid function tests show that she is hypothyroid.

The most common cause of hypothyroidism is Hashimoto's thyroiditis, in which thyroid follicular cells are destroyed by the immune system. Which molecule, secreted by cytotoxic T-cells, results in thyroid follicular cell apoptosis?

A  IFN-$\gamma$
B  TNF-$\alpha$
C  Fas ligand
D  Granzyme
E  Perforin

10. A 14-year-old girl has presented to her GP with a rash on her neck. There is a clearly defined 4 cm × 2 cm erythematous patch over her sternal notch. She mentions that she has been wearing a necklace that her mother recently gave her.
    Which immune cell is most likely implicated in this response?

    A  IgE secreting plasma cells
    B  IgG secreting plasma cells
    C  Mast cells
    D  Basophils
    E  T-helper I cells

11. By what receptor-mediated process do neutrophils exit the circulation to a site of infection?

    A  Extravasation
    B  Chemotaxis
    C  Rolling
    D  Exudation
    E  Diapedesis

12. Chédiak-Higashi syndrome is a rare autosomal recessive disorder that impairs lysosomal function in immune cells.
    Which of the following processes is likely to be affected by this disease?

    **A** Antibody secretion
    **B** Cytokine release
    **C** Cytotoxic response
    **D** Phagocytosis
    **E** Complement pathway

13. Which enzyme enables bacteriophages to be released from a host cell?

    **A** Neuraminidase
    **B** Reverse transcriptase
    **C** Integrase
    **D** Lysins
    **E** Hemagglutinin esterase

14. A 51-year-old man is recovering in ITU after developing acute respiratory distress syndrome (ARDS). Significant necrosis of type I pneumocytes is typically seen in ARDS.
What molecule, released by necrotic cells, can stimulate the innate immune system?

    **A** Hyaluronan
    **B** Mitochondrial ATP
    **C** Defensins
    **D** Fibrinogen
    **E** ssRNA

15. A 23-year-old woman with a background of juvenile idiopathic arthritis has presented with a high fever, coagulopathy and a low cell count. This is thought to be a complication of her known diagnosis of macrophage activation syndrome.
Which of the following cytokines is primarily involved in activating macrophages?

    **A** IFN-$\gamma$
    **B** TGF-$\beta$

    **C** TNF-$\alpha$
    **D** IL8
    **E** IL12

16. A 31-year-old man has become jaundiced and feverish after returning from a trip to South East Asia. He had drunkenly got a tattoo on his right buttock and is unsure about whether a clean needle was used. Viral hepatitis is suspected, and an antibody screen is requested.
    The presence of raised levels of which of the following types of antibody would you expect to see during an acute infection?

    **A** IgG
    **B** IgM
    **C** IgA
    **D** IgD
    **E** IgE

17. Which endothelial molecule do naïve T-cells tightly bind to during lymph node migration?

    **A** ICAM-I
    **B** LFA-I
    **C** L-Selectin
    **D** CD34
    **E** Glycam-I

18. A 44-year-old man with HIV is being treated for *Pneumocystis* pneumonia with a course of co-trimoxazole. This combination antibiotic contains sulfamethoxazole which is a sulfonamide.
    Which of the following is a known mechanism of resistance to sulfonamide antibiotics?

    **A** Altered target site
    **B** Methylation of 50S ribosome
    **C** Drug efflux pumps

**D** Beta-lactamase production

**E** Increased production of PABA

19. Which of the following cytokines has an anti-inflammatory effect?

    **A** IFN-$\gamma$

    **B** IL5

    **C** IL8

    **D** IL10

    **E** IL17

20. What function is performed by C3b complement in the classical pathway?

    **A** Promotes inflammation

    **B** Formation of membrane attack complex

    **C** Opsonisation

    **D** Neutrophil recruitment

    **E** Activation of C3 convertase

21. Which immune cell type is primarily affected by HIV?

    **A** Cytotoxic T-cells

    **B** T-helper cells

    **C** B cells

    **D** Monocytes

    **E** Natural killer cells

22. *Staphylococcus* is described as a catalase-positive bacterium. How does this feature support their survival?

    **A** Sequestration of antibody

    **B** Inhibition of chemotaxis

    **C** Stimulation of inhibitory immune receptors

    **D** Neutralisation of reactive oxygen species

    **E** Lysis of leukocytes

23. Which of the following diseases will mainly affect the innate immune response?

    **A** Acute myeloid leukaemia
    **B** B cell lymphoma
    **C** AIRE mutation
    **D** Adenosine deaminase deficiency
    **E** HIV

24. A 27-year-old man has presented to his sexual health clinic with a painful rash on his penis. On examination, there is a discrete cluster of tender vesicles on the shaft of his penis.
Which medication is most likely to be prescribed?

    **A** Azidothymidine
    **B** Oseltamivir
    **C** Amantadine
    **D** Baloxavir
    **E** Acyclovir

25. A 54-year-old man has developed a continuous high fever and a severe headache. He has also developed multiple bruises across his arms. He lives in a rural part of Brazil which has a high incidence of dengue. He had dengue earlier this year, however, his symptoms were considerably milder.
Which of the following would explain the increased severity of the symptoms he is experiencing?

    **A** Viral mutation resulting in increased virulence
    **B** Antibody-dependent enhancement of different viral serotypes
    **C** Suppression of antibody production
    **D** Virus secretes surface antigens that evade antibody detection
    **E** Antigenic shift of virus

26. A 57-year-old woman has been admitted to the general medical ward with suspected community-acquired pneumonia. She is started on IV

co-amoxiclav. Within 10 minutes, her breathing becomes noisy, her oxygen saturations drop and she develops a widespread rash.
Which of the following mechanisms underpins this clinical scenario?

A IgE cross-linking on mast cells
B Opsonisation of penicillin-antigen complex
C Presentation of penicillin antigens to sensitised T-cells
D Cross-reactivity of anti-penicillin antibodies with host cell antigens
E Lysis of bacteria releases proinflammatory mediators

27. What is the bacterial target of vancomycin?

A DNA gyrase
B 50S ribosomal subunit
C Cell wall
D Cell membrane
E RNA polymerase

28. How do B-cell receptors achieve sufficient variability in their antigen specificity?

A Variable region determines antibody type
B Somatic hypermutation in Peyer's patches
C VDJ recombination of heavy and light chains
D MHC-II and TCR interactions
E Polysaccharide epitopes binding to B-cell receptors

29. A defect in NADPH oxidase results in a reduction in the generation of reactive oxygen species.
What immunodeficiency is most likely to be a consequence of this defect?

A Leukocyte adhesion deficiency
B Chronic granulomatous disease

    **C** Severe combined immunodeficiency
    **D** Agammaglobulinemia
    **E** Complement deficiency

30. Which soluble mediator of innate immunity recognises carbohydrate patterns on the surface of pathogenic microorganisms?

    **A** Complement
    **B** Acute phase proteins
    **C** Mannose-binding lectin
    **D** Leukotrienes
    **E** Reactive oxygen species

31. Which of the following cytokines and corresponding cells would be primarily involved in the immune response to a tapeworm infection?

    **A** IFN-$\gamma$ by Th1 cells
    **B** TNF-$\alpha$ by CD8 cells
    **C** IL5 by Th2 cells
    **D** IL17 by Th17 cells
    **E** IL21 by Tfh cells

32. A 42-year-old woman has presented with a vague history of lethargy, weight loss and muscle weakness. Her 9 am cortisol is noted to be low and a short synacthen test confirms a diagnosis of primary adrenal insufficiency, likely secondary to T-cell-mediated autoimmune attack.
   Which of the following mechanisms involves controlling self-reactive T-cells by inactivation?

    **A** Conversion to T-regulatory cells
    **B** Apoptosis
    **C** Negative selection
    **D** Immunological ignorance
    **E** Induction of anergy

33. Which of the following is a mechanism by which bacteria can acquire antibiotic resistance via a bacteriophage?

    A  Bacterial transformation
    B  Bacterial transposons
    C  Bacterial conjugation
    D  Bacterial transduction
    E  Horizontal gene transfer

34. Through which molecule does SARS-CoV-2 enter type II pneumocytes?

    A  Sialic acid receptor
    B  Glycosaminoglycans in IGF 1 receptor
    C  ICAM-I
    D  ACE-II
    E  CAR

35. A 44-year-old tea plucker in the Sri Lankan hill country is bitten by a venomous snake and antivenom is promptly administered. This has happened on one previous occasion in which she was treated success-fully with antivenom. On this occasion, however, she develops a fever, rash and generalised body pain a week after receiving treatment for her snake bite.
    What is the most likely reason for this reaction?

    A  Exaggerated IgM response to venom
    B  Deposition of IgG-venom immune complexes in joints
    C  Delayed T-cell-mediated cellular response to venom
    D  Host antibodies directed against antivenom antibodies
    E  Antivenom has not recognised this type of snake venom

36. The activation of B-cells by T-cells requires a costimulatory signal between which of the following cell surface receptors?

    A  CD28 and B7
    B  MHC-II and CD4

    **C** MHC-I and CD8

    **D** CD40 and CD40L

    **E** CTLA-4 and B7

37. Enfuvirtide is a drug used in the treatment of HIV. It targets the gp41 transmembrane glycoprotein and prevents it from penetrating the cell membrane.

    Which of the following best describes this type of antiviral drug?

    **A** Protease inhibitor

    **B** Integrase inhibitor

    **C** Fusion inhibitor

    **D** Non-nucleoside reverse transcriptase inhibitor

    **E** Co-receptor antagonist

38. Which cell surface marker is downregulated in virus-infected cells?

    **A** PDL-1

    **B** MHC-I

    **C** MHC-II

    **D** CD45

    **E** FAS

39. A 62-year-old man with a background of alcohol excess is admitted onto the acute medical unit after developing a high fever and a productive cough. It started 2 days ago and he has been bringing up large volumes of purulent sputum. A chest X-ray reveals multiple patchy opacities in the right lung with a cavitating lesion within the right middle zone.

    Which of the following organisms is most likely to have led to this condition?

    **A** *Klebsiella pneumoniae*

    **B** *Haemophilus influenzae*

    **C** *Mycobacterium tuberculosis*

  **D** *Legionella pneumophila*
  **E** *Mycoplasma pneumoniae*

40. A 42-year-old man has become unwell over the past 4 days with a high fever, headaches and joint pain. This began after he went on a holiday to the Cotswolds which involved several long walks through the countryside. On examination, a target-shaped red rash is seen on his back. He is diagnosed with Lyme disease and started on a course of doxycycline. An hour after taking his first dose of doxycycline, his fever gets worse, he begins to hyperventilate and becomes tachycardic.
   What is the most likely cause of the worsening of his symptoms?

  **A** Serum sickness
  **B** Bacterial cell death
  **C** Anaphylaxis
  **D** Antibody dependent enhancement
  **E** Inflammatory cell margination

## Answers

### 1. B (Type II hypersensitivity)

Haemolytic disease of the newborn is an important neonatal condition that is caused by the presence of maternal anti-D antibodies which result in the destruction of foetal red cells. This can cause jaundice and profound anaemia. The Rhesus D (RhD) antigen is an important antigen that is found on the surface of red cells and is inherited in an autosomal dominant manner. The 'positive' that is stated in blood grouping refers to the presence of the RhD antigen. RhD antigen differs from the A and B antigens in that those who are negative for RhD antigen do not have naturally occurring antibodies against RhD. The child from this patient's first pregnancy may have been RhD positive. This would have been recognised as foreign by the maternal immune system. During her first pregnancy, IgM antibodies would have been produced which cannot cross the placenta — therefore, the firstborn child is unaffected. During the second pregnancy, exposure to RhD-positive blood from the foetus will trigger an IgG-mediated response resulting in the binding of antibodies to RhD antigens on foetal red cells. This results in widespread red cell haemolysis. This is an example of a type II hypersensitivity reaction, which is caused by the binding of antibodies against cellular or extracellular matrix antigens.

Type I hypersensitivity is characterised by the IgE-mediated release of histamine from mast cells and basophils. This results in an acute inflammatory response (anaphylaxis). Type III hypersensitivity is caused by the failure of clearance of antigen-antibody immune complexes. This can result in inflammation and tissue damage. Rheumatoid arthritis and SLE are examples of type III hypersensitivity reactions. Type IV hypersensitivity is characterised by a delayed T-cell mediated response with an initial sensitisation phase in which the antigen is presented to naive T-cells by antigen-presenting cells. Subsequent exposure to the same antigen triggered a T-cell mediated inflammatory response that tends to be most evident 2–3 days after exposure. Type V hypersensitivity refers to the production of antibodies that are capable of stimulating certain targets (e.g. TSH-receptor stimulating antibodies in Graves' disease).

## 2. C (Neutrophil)

Acute inflammation is defined as the vascular and tissue response to cellular injury. It results in the recruitment of inflammatory cells to the site of injury. Neutrophils are the first responders to a site of acute inflammation. They are able to phagocytose cell debris and pathogens and release various cytokines that promote the recruitment of other inflammatory cells (e.g. macrophages). A biopsy of acutely inflamed tissue will reveal an abundance of neutrophils.

Macrophages also play an important role in phagocytosis; however, they are present in fewer numbers in acutely inflamed tissue. Eosinophils are implicated in allergic responses and immune responses to parasites. Mast cells contain histamine and have IgE on their cell membranes. The cross-linking of IgE by allergens results in mast cell degranulation. CD8+ T-cells are cytotoxic T-cells that kill virus-infected or malignant cells.

## 3. D (T-regulatory cell)

T-regulatory cells (CD4+CD25+) are responsible for regulating the effector and activation stages of T-cells. They inhibit other types of T-cells, thereby suppressing the immune response. This is a component of peripheral tolerance that prevents autoimmune disease. Foxp3 is a transcription factor that is important in the differentiation and function of T-regulatory cells. Therefore, a Foxp3 mutation results in dysfunction of immune surveillance and peripheral tolerance, thereby resulting in autoimmune disease.

## 4. C (Macrolides)

Atypical pneumonia, as the name suggests, is characterised by an atypical presentation. Rather than presenting with a classical productive cough and a fever, they may present with malaise, myalgia, dry cough, diarrhoea and confusion. The main causes of atypical pneumonia are *Legionella pneumophila*, *Mycoplasma pneumoniae* and *Chlamydia pneumoniae*. Macrolides (e.g. clarithromycin) are very effective at treating atypical pneumonia. They work by targeting the 50S ribosomal subunit and preventing amino-acyl transfer. This results in an inability to form peptide bonds between adjacent amino acids during translation. The inability to synthesise proteins results in suppression of bacterial growth.

Aminoglycosides (e.g. gentamicin) are bactericidal. They target the 30S ribosomal subunit thereby impairing protein synthesis. Fluoroquinolones (e.g. ciprofloxacin) are bactericidal antibiotics that target DNA gyrase. This prevents the unfolding of bacterial DNA, thereby resulting in impaired cell division. Fluoroquinolones are particularly effective against Gram-negative organisms. Cephalosporins (e.g. ceftriaxone) are a class of beta-lactam antibiotics which, similarly to penicillins, inhibit the formation of a peptidoglycan cell wall. Glycopeptides (e.g. vancomycin) also prevent the formation of the peptidoglycan cell wall. They are particularly effective against Gram-positive bacteria (e.g. *C. difficile*).

## 5. B (Bone marrow)

Immature B-cells present in the bone marrow will undergo a process called VDJ recombination which enables the production of a huge variety of B-cell receptors. It is achieved by the action of VDJ recombinase which alters the order of V, D and J exon regions within the primary lymphoid organs (bone marrow for B-cells and thymus gland for T-cells). Secondary lymphoid organs such as the spleen, Peyer's patches and lymph nodes are locations where lymphocytes can interact with antigens and other lymphocytes.

## 6. D (Mononuclear cell infiltrate)

Granulomatous inflammation is a form of chronic inflammation in which aggregates of activated macrophages and lymphocytes (granuloma) form a barrier around a perceived foreign threat. This aims to prevent the spread of infection and is usually seen in tuberculosis (TB). Sarcoidosis is an autoimmune disease of unknown aetiology characterised by the formation of granulomas in various tissues across the body without any primary insult (i.e. it is like the immune response to TB without the bacteria being present). Granulomatous inflammation can result in fibrosis.

## 7. A (PDL-I)

Programmed cell death protein I (PDL-I) and CD279 are cell-surface proteins that downregulate T-cells and promote self-tolerance. Malignant cells can express large quantities of PDL-I thereby enabling the tumour to evade immune surveillance.

B7 is a costimulatory protein expressed on the surface of antigen-presenting cells which interacts with CD28 on T-cells. FAS ligand is a transmembrane protein that can induce apoptosis within a cell by binding to the FAS ligand. Autoimmune regulator (AIRE) is a transcription factor that enables the expression of a variety of host proteins within the thymus gland, with which self-reactive T-cells can be negatively selected before leaving the thymus. This is a form of central immune tolerance. A mutation in AIRE will result in autoimmune polyendocrinopathy candidiasis ectodermal dystrophy (APECED). p53 is a tumour-suppressor protein encoded by the TP53 gene. It has a number of functions, including DNA repair, apoptosis and regulating the cell cycle. Mutating and disabling the TP53 gene can increase the risk of uncontrolled cell division and, hence, cancer.

## 8. B (Protein A)

Protein A, expressed on the surface of *Staphylococcus aureus*, binds to the Fc portion of antibodies and inhibits opsonisation. This means that *S. aureus* can evade detection and destruction by phagocytes.

Staphylococcal complement inhibitor (SCIN) inhibits complement-mediated phagocytosis. Factor H is another protein that can reduce complement activity. Chemotaxis inhibitory proteins are exoproteins secreted by *S. aureus* which inhibit the chemotaxis of neutrophils and monocytes, thereby impeding the recruitment of inflammatory cells to the site of infection. Staphylococcal superantigen-like protein 7 (SSL7) inhibits complement by preventing the formation of the membrane attack complex.

## 9. D (Granzyme)

Hashimoto's thyroiditis is a condition in which autoimmune destruction of thyroid follicular cells results in hypothyroidism. As thyroid hormone is important in maintaining the body's metabolic rate, hypothyroidism manifests with features of 'slowing down' such as lethargy, constipation, depression and weight gain. There are a number of autoantibodies that may be produced in Hashimoto's thyroiditis such as anti-thyroid peroxidase and anti-thyroglobulin antibodies. The aberrant recognition of thyroid follicular cells as foreign results in a cytotoxic CD8 response. These cells release perforin and granzymes which results in the apoptotic death of thyroid follicular cells. Perforin binds to the membrane of the target cells and forms a pore, which allows granzymes to enter and trigger apoptosis.

IFN-$\gamma$ is a proinflammatory cytokine that activates macrophages. TNF-$\alpha$ is a proinflammatory cytokine produced by macrophages. Activated CD8+ cells express Fas ligand on their cell surface. It binds to Fas receptors on target cells and the Fas-FasL interaction triggers an intracellular caspase cascade which, eventually, results in cell death. Perforin is released with granzyme during a cytotoxic T-cell response. Perforin inserts itself into the membrane and forms pores through which granzyme can enter the cell and cause apoptosis.

## 10. E (T-helper I cells)

A type IV hypersensitivity reaction is a delayed form of allergic response in which there is an initial sensitisation phase. During this phase, allergens are presented to naive T-cells by antigen-presenting cells. Upon subsequent exposure, the same antigen will be presented to Th1 cells by antigen-presenting cells thereby triggering an inflammatory response. In the context of contact dermatitis, it manifests as swelling and redness in the area of skin that made direct contact with the allergen.

IgE cross-linking in type I hypersensitivity reactions results in mast cell degranulation and an acute inflammatory response. IgG immunoglobulins directed at cellular antigens is the basis of type II hypersensitivity reactions. Mast cells release histamine in response to IgE cross-linking in type I hypersensitivity reactions. Basophils are also implicated in type I hypersensitivity reactions.

## 11. E (Diapedesis)

Neutrophil migration to a site of injury results from the release of IL8 from macrophages, which upregulates endothelial adhesion molecules (selectins). Rolling and adhesion occurs as neutrophils first establish reversible binding between selectins on the endothelial surface and carbohydrate ligands. Tight adhesion to endothelial cells is mediated by interactions between MAC-I and LFA-I present on neutrophils and ICAM-1 and ICAM-2 ligands on the endothelial surface. Once fixed, the neutrophils will migrate across the endothelium along a chemotactic gradient. The movement of neutrophils from the circulation into the tissues is called diapedesis.

## 12. D (Phagocytosis)

Chediak-Higashi syndrome is an inherited and rare autosomal recessive disorder that is characterised by immunodeficiency due to a mutation of a lysosomal trafficking regulator protein. This impairs the migration and function of lysosomes within granulocytes. The action of lysosomes is essential for the phagocytosis and digestion of pathogens. A lysosomal defect, therefore, will impede the function of phagocytes.

## 13. D (Lysins)

Lysins are hydrolytic enzymes that are synthesised by bacteriophages using the machinery of host cells. They target the peptidoglycan cell wall and enable bacteriophage exit from the host cell.

Neuraminidase cleaves sialic acid residues on the surface of cells and prevents them from binding to haemagglutinin on the surface of viruses that are being produced by the cells. Neuraminidase inhibitors (e.g. oseltamivir) can, therefore, prevent the release of influenza from host cells. Reverse transcriptase is an enzyme that is produced by retroviruses and is able to reverse transcribe positive sense RNA into dsDNA. Integrase is an enzyme expressed by retroviruses that can integrate the dsDNA produced by reverse transcription into the host DNA. Haemagglutinin esterase is an enzyme produced by influenza which destroys sialic acid receptors on the membrane of host cells.

## 14.  B (Mitochondrial ATP)

Necrotic cells release damage associated molecular patterns (DAMPs) which can be detected by toll-like receptors on the surface of macrophages. Mitochondrial ATP is not typically found within the extracellular environment, so detection of this molecule is suggestive of cellular damage and will trigger an innate immune response.

Hyaluronan is an extracellular matrix protein that is released due to damage to the basement membrane by neutrophil proteases in acute lung injury. It can also be detected by toll-like receptors; however, it does not result from necrosis of type I pneumocytes. Defensins are released by macrophages, neutrophils and Paneth cells. Fibrinogen is the precursor of fibrin that is found within the bloodstream. A low level of fibrinogen is seen in disseminated intravascular coagulation due to increased consumption of clotting factors. ssRNA is a form of pathogen-associated molecular pattern produced by viruses.

## 15.  A (IFN-$\gamma$)

IFN-$\gamma$ is released by several immune cells, such as Th1 cells which are the primary activators of macrophages. The activation of macrophages by IFN-$\gamma$ enhances their phagocytic capabilities.

TGF-$\beta$ is an anti-inflammatory cytokine released by T regulatory cells. They suppress macrophage activity. TNF-$\alpha$ is a proinflammatory cytokine predominantly released by activated macrophages. IL8 is a chemotactic cytokine that enables the recruitment of neutrophils to the site of injury.

IL12 is a proinflammatory cytokine secreted by dendritic cells and macrophages which enhances the cytotoxic effects of NK cells and CD8+ T-cells.

## 16. B (IgM)

In the initial response to viral infection, IgM antibodies are secreted by B-cells. As a general principle, the presence of high titres of the IgM form of an antibody directed against a particular virus (e.g. hepatitis B) is suggestive of an acute infection. Following the acute phase, there is a class switch in antibody production. Maintenance of immunity against a particular antigen is achieved by the production of IgG antibodies. The presence of high titres of IgG antibodies and absence of IgM is suggestive of previous infection or vaccination. IgA antibodies are usually found on mucosal surfaces (e.g. gastrointestinal tract). IgD antibodies are found in low concentrations and their function is poorly defined. IgE antibodies are involved in allergy and responses to parasitic infections.

## 17. A (ICAM-I)

Naïve T-cells access lymph nodes from the circulation via specialised blood vessels called high endothelial venules (HEV). Naïve T-cells express CCR7 receptors and adhesions molecules (L-selectin and LFA-I). L-selectin facilitates the rolling of the cells along the endothelial cells in the HEV. Cells within the lymph node express CCL21 which binds to CCR7 on the naïve T-cells and induces a conformational change in the LFA-1 molecule. This results in LFA-I binding more tightly to ICAM-I. This arrests the T-cell along the endothelium which then allows the movement of the cell into the lymph node (diapedesis).

## 18. E (Increased production of PABA)

Sulfonamide antibiotics are structural analogues of para-aminobenzoic acid (PABA) which is an intermediate in folic acid synthesis. Folic acid is an essential component of DNA synthesis. Bacteria can become resistant to sulfonamides by increasing their production of PABA such that the

substrate outcompetes the sulfonamide antibiotic, thereby enabling sufficient folic acid synthesis for DNA replication.

Methicillin-resistant *Staphylococcus aureus* (MRSA) encodes an altered
PBP2a (target of penicillin) which has a low affinity for beta-lactam antibiotics. This is an example of an altered target site as a mechanism of
antibiotic resistance. *Streptococcus pneumoniae* resistance to erythromycin occurs via the acquisition of the erm gene, which encodes an enzyme
that methylates the 50S ribosomal subunit thereby preventing the binding
of erythromycin. Drug efflux pumps can be used by bacteria to prevent the
accumulation of antibiotics in their intracellular environment. This mechanism has been seen in *Staphylococcus aureus*. Beta-lactamases are
enzymes produced by bacteria (e.g. *E. coli*) which hydrolyse the beta-
lactam ring within the structure of penicillin, thus rendering it
ineffective.

## 19.  D (IL10)

IL10 is a pleiotropic anti-inflammatory cytokine that is predominantly
produced by monocytes and T-regulatory cells. It downregulates macrophage activity by inhibiting the synthesis of proinflammatory cytokines.

IFN-$\gamma$ is a proinflammatory cytokine primarily secreted by natural killer
cells and activated T-cells. It promotes macrophage activation. IL5 is a
mediator of eosinophil maturation and is implicated in the pathophysiology of asthma. IL8 is a neutrophil chemoattractant that is released by
activated macrophages in response to tissue injury. IL17 is a proinflammatory cytokine that is released by Th17 cells. It also promotes the chemotaxis of neutrophils.

## 20.  C (Opsonisation)

The complement system is a system of proteins that 'complements' the
clearance of pathogens and cell debris by antibodies and phagocytes.
There are two pathways of complement activation: classical and alternative. The classical pathway is triggered by antibody binding to an antigen,

whereas the alternative pathway is triggered by direct binding of complement components to microbial proteins. Both the classical and alternative pathways result in the activation of C3 convertase. This then leads to the splitting of C3 into C3a (involved in inflammation) and C3b (involved in opsonisation). There is a third pathway of complement activation, which is less physiologically significant, known as the lectin pathway.

### 21. B (T-helper cells)

The HIV replication cycle involves the attachment of the viral Env glycoprotein spike to the T-helper cell surface receptor, CD4, and co-receptor, CCR5. This can lead to T-helper cell depletion and immunodeficiency.

Cytotoxic T-cells express CD8. They release cytotoxic granules (perforin and granzyme) that can kill virus-infected and malignant cells. B-cells are responsible for the humoral immune system. They differentiate into antibody-secreting plasma cells and memory cells. 'Monocyte' is the term used to describe macrophages before they leave the circulation to enter tissues. They have a role in presenting antigens to lymphocytes and they develop into macrophages to execute phagocytic functions. Natural killer cells are part of the innate immune response. They recognise 'non-self' and, hence, are involved in the identification and destruction of virus-infected and tumour cells.

### 22. D (Neutralisation of reactive oxygen species)

Catalase is an enzyme produced by some bacteria which breaks down hydrogen peroxide and neutralises reactive oxygen species that are secreted by neutrophils. This protects them from inflammatory cell-mediated oxidative damage.

### 23. A (Acute myeloid leukaemia)

Acute myeloid leukaemia is a bone marrow malignancy characterised by an excessive production of dysfunctional myeloblasts. Due to a failure of maturation, this results in a decrease in the total number of functional granulocytes, which are part of the innate immune system. The predominance of one aberrant clone of myeloblasts results in the crowding out of other blood cell precursors from the bone marrow. This leads to pancytopaenia (anaemia, leukopaenia and thrombocytopaenia). Therefore, acute myeloid leukaemia is likely to end up affecting both innate and adaptive immunity.

B-cell lymphomas can affect B-cell function, which is a component of the adaptive immune system. B-cells differentiate into antibody-secreting plasma cells or memory cells. AIRE (autoimmune regulator) is a transcription factor that enables the expression of a panel of self-antigens within the thymus. Self-reactive T-cells can then be negatively selected against this panel. A defect in the AIRE gene results in Autoimmune Polyendocrinopathy Candidiasis Ectodermal Dystrophy, which is characterised by a failure of central tolerance. Adenosine deaminase deficiency is an autosomal recessive condition that results in severe combined immunodeficiency. HIV targets CD4+ T-helper cells resulting in lymphopenia and, hence, a defective adaptive immune response.

### 24. E (Acyclovir)

Acyclovir is an antiviral that is commonly used to treat herpes simplex virus infections. It is an analogue of 2' deoxyguanosine and acts as a chain terminator. Acyclovir is administered in an inactive form that requires viral thymidine kinase (produced only within herpes-infected cells) to phosphorylate acyclovir into acycloguanosine monophosphate. Two further phosphorylation steps will produce acycloguanosine triphosphate, which is the active form of acyclovir. This ensures that acyclovir only acts as a DNA chain terminator in cells that are infected by herpes simplex virus.

Azidothymidine (zidovudine) is a nucleotide analogue of thymidine. It competitively inhibits reverse transcriptase and is used in the treatment of HIV. Oseltamivir is a competitive inhibitor of the viral neuraminidase enzyme. It prevents the release of influenza virus from infected host cells. Amantadine interacts with the transmembrane domain of the M2 protein of the virus. The virus enters the host cell through receptor-mediated endocytosis. Once within the vesicle, acidification occurs via the passage of hydrogen ions through the M2 ion channel. This releases the viral machinery into the cell. Baloxavir inhibits the endonuclease function of RNA-dependent polymerase. This prevents RNA replication.

## 25. B (Antibody-dependent enhancement of different viral serotypes)

Dengue virus is a mosquito-borne virus that is prevalent in many tropical countries. It typically presents with fever and myalgia. There are four main serotypes of dengue virus. When someone is infected by dengue, they will produce antibodies against that particular serotype of dengue virus. Upon subsequent exposure to a different serotype of dengue virus, these antibodies can bind to the virus, however, they cannot neutralise it. The antibody binding, in fact, helps the virus to infect monocytes and cause more severe disease. This is known as antibody-dependent enhancement.

## 26. A (IgE cross-linking on mast cells)

This vignette is describing a patient having an anaphylactic reaction to co-amoxiclav. This is a type I hypersensitivity reaction which is mediated by the cross-linking of IgE on the surface of mast cells. This results in mast cell degranulation, releasing large amounts of histamines which have a profound proinflammatory effect. Features of anaphylaxis include airway compromise (due to laryngeal oedema) and urticaria.

Opsonisation of penicillin-antigen complexes would be an example of a type II hypersensitivity reaction. Penicillin can cause this (and all other) type of hypersensitivity reactions; however, the presentation is more suggestive of anaphylaxis. Presentation of an antigen to sensitised T-cells is the mechanism by which type IV hypersensitivity occurs. Antibody cross-reactivity refers to the phenomenon by which an antibody directed against a particular antigen mistakenly binds to a similar-looking antigen. This can occur in certain pathological states, such as rheumatic heart disease, in which antibodies directed against streptococcal antigens cross-react with antigens on heart valves. The lysis of bacteria following antibiotic treatment can result in the release of various endotoxins that can trigger a systemic inflammatory response. This is known as a Jarisch–Herxheimer reaction and it is usually associated with the treatment of syphilis.

### 27.  C (Cell wall)

Vancomycin is a glycopeptide antibiotic that works by inhibiting bacterial cell wall synthesis. It prevents the synthesis of polymers of N-acetylmuramic acid (NAM) and N-acetylglucosamine (NAG) which form the backbone of the cell wall. It is mainly effective against Gram-positive bacteria and is widely used in the treatment of *C. difficile*.

DNA gyrase is responsible for unravelling DNA in the process of cell division. It is the target of fluoroquinolone antibiotics. The 50S ribosomal subunit is the target of macrolides. The cell membrane is the target of daptomycin. RNA polymerase is the target of rifampicin which is used in the treatment of tuberculosis.

### 28.  C (VDJ recombination of heavy and light chains)

Maturing B-cells within the bone marrow will undergo VDJ recombination in order to produce a sufficiently varied population of B-cell receptors. VDJ recombinase will rearrange the V, D and J exon regions to produce distinct B-cell receptors. This occurs within primary lymphoid organs.

The constant region determines the type of antibody and is formed by heavy chains only. Peyer's patches are areas of lymphoid tissue that are located within the gastrointestinal mucosa. B-cells may migrate to such secondary lymphoid organs to undergo somatic hypermutation. This is a process by which the antibody response to a certain antigen increases in affinity. Following antigen detection by the B-cell receptor, the antigen will be endocytosed and processed before being presented via MHC-II to

CD4+ T-helper cells. This triggers the release of cytokines that promote B-cell differentiation into plasma cells. Polysaccharides contain repeating subunits that can bind to B-cell receptors which, in the presence of a secondary signal by other pathogen-associated molecular patterns, can activate B-cells.

### 29. B (Chronic granulomatous disease)

Chronic granulomatous disease is a primary immunodeficiency caused by a defect in the NADPH oxidase complex within neutrophils. NADPH oxidase generates superoxide species to neutralise pathogens during phagocytosis. Defective NADPH oxidase function, therefore, will result in an inability to generate superoxide and, hence, inflict oxidative damage on pathogens. This, in turn, results in increased susceptibility to infection. Repeated inflammation results in granuloma formation.

Leukocyte adhesion deficiency is an autosomal recessive disorder caused by defects in integrin function. This leads to impaired chemotaxis and immune cell recruitment to sites of injury. Severe combined immunodeficiency is a condition in which the development of both B and T-cells is impaired. There are a number of causes such as adenosine deaminase deficiency. Agammaglobulinemia refers to reduced serum immunoglobulin levels leading to defects in humoral immunity. Complement deficiency can be primary (inherited) or acquired (secondary to systemic lupus erythematosus). It can result in increased susceptibility to infection.

### 30. C (Mannose-binding lectin)

Mannose-binding lectins are soluble mediators of the innate immune system. They recognise carbohydrate patterns on the surface of microorganisms, resulting in complement activation. This is called the lectin pathway of complement activation, which plays a relatively minor physiological role compared to the classical and alternative pathways of complement activation. A deficiency in mannose-binding lectin can lead to an increased risk of infection.

Complement is a system of plasma proteins that 'complement' the opsonisation and destruction of bacteria by phagocytes and antibodies. There are three pathways of complement activation (classical, alternative and lectin) which converge on the C3 protein. C3 activation will result in the formation of a membrane attack complex. Acute phase proteins are serum markers that change in concentration during acute inflammatory states. Examples include C reactive protein, ferritin and albumin. Leukotrienes are inflammatory cytokines that are produced by the arachidonic acid pathway. They can cause several deleterious effects such as bronchoconstriction. Reactive oxygen species are free radicals that are released by inflammatory cells. They can cause cell death by inflicting oxidative damage.

### 31. C (IL5 by Th2 cells)

Tapeworms are parasites that induce an inflammatory response mediated by Th2 cells. Dendritic cells within the gastrointestinal mucosa present antigens of the parasite to T-cells, thereby resulting in T-cell activation. Th2 cells then release IL4, IL5 and IL12 which facilitates the recruitment of inflammatory cells. The inflammatory response to parasitic infections usually involves an abundance of IgE-producing B-cells, mast cells and eosinophils.

### 32. E (Induction of anergy)

Peripheral tolerance is an immunological mechanism by which self-reactive lymphocytes are neutralised in order to prevent autoimmune reactions. The activation of naive T-cells requires the presence of costimulatory signals which are normally stimulated by proinflammatory cytokines. The presentation of a self-antigen to a T-cell without costimulatory signals will promote a state of inactivity (anergy).

Self-reactive T-cells can be suppressed by being converted into T regulatory cells. Apoptosis of self-reactive T-cells can be induced via FAS-FAS ligand interactions. Negative selection is an example of central tolerance within the thymus gland. The autoimmune regulator (AIRE) gene encodes a special transcription factor that can express various self-proteins within the thymus gland, thereby creating a panel of self-antigens against which immature T-cells can be tested. Self-reactive T-cells can then be negatively selected (i.e. destroyed). Immunological ignorance is the term used to describe the inability of self-reactive T-cells to reach certain immunologically privileged sites (e.g. eyes).

### 33.  D (Bacterial transduction)

Lysogenic bacteriophages can pick up bacterial DNA encoding genes for antibiotic resistance. When the bacteriophage infects a subsequent bacterium, it can integrate this resistance gene into the bacterial host's genome. This is known as bacterial transduction.

Bacterial transformation is a process by which bacterial cells take up DNA fragments from their surrounding environment, some of which may confer antibiotic resistance. Bacterial transposons are segments of DNA that can be exchanged and integrated between bacterial genomes. Bacterial conjugation involves the exchange of bacterial plasmids through a non-contact process. Adjacent bacteria can create a tubular connection (pilus) through which plasmids encoding resistance genes can be passed. Horizontal gene transfer is a broad term defining the process in which genetic material is exchanged between bacteria.

### 34.  D (ACE-II)

The SARS-CoV-2 spike protein binds to ACE-II receptors expressed by type II pneumocytes within the respiratory epithelium. This binding enables viral entry into host cells.

Haemagglutinin on the surface of influenza binds to sialic acid receptors in the upper respiratory tract. F and G proteins of respiratory syncytial virus bind to glycosaminoglycan in IGFR1 and nucleolin receptors. The human rhinovirus binds to ICAM-I on the surface of respiratory epithelial cells. Adenovirus C-fibres bind onto CAR, allowing viral attachment to the cell surface.

### 35. D (Host antibodies directed against antivenom antibodies)

Serum sickness is a type III hypersensitivity reaction in which the immune system recognises exogenously administered proteins (such as antivenom) as foreign and develops an antibody response against them. The first time they are exposed to these 'foreign' proteins is the sensitisation phase in which the immune system learns to recognise the protein as foreign. This does not usually cause any clinical manifestations. The second time the immune system encounters the protein, however, will result in an immune complex-mediated response in which host antibodies bind to the antivenom, resulting in complement activation and inflammation. It usually presents about 5–10 days after exposure and manifests with vague symptoms such as fever, malaise and arthralgia.

### 36. D (CD40 and CD40L)

The T-cell receptor on CD4+ T-cells can bind to MHC-II on B-cells and affect their function. The type of interaction that occurs depends on the costimulatory signal. An interaction between CD40 on B-cells and CD40 ligands on T-cells relays a costimulatory signal that promotes the differentiation of B-cells into plasma cells.

### 37. C (Fusion inhibitor)

The HIV replication cycle begins with the attachment of viral gp120 to CD4 receptors on T-helper cells. This induces a conformational change resulting in the binding of co-receptors (CCR5). The expression of gp41 by the virus enables the penetration of the lymphocyte membrane and, hence, enabling fusion between the HIV virions and the host cell. By targeting gp41, it prevents fusion.

Virally encoded proteases are responsible for the cleavage of various protein components of HIV that are necessary for viral replication. Integrase inhibitors (e.g. dolutegravir) prevents the insertion of HIV DNA into the host genome. Non-Nucleoside Reverse Transcriptase Inhibitors (NNRTI) non-competitively inhibits reverse transcriptase enzymes, thereby preventing the formation of dsDNA. Co-receptor antagonists (e.g. maraviroc) inhibit the CCR5 co-receptor from binding onto the HIV glycoproteins, thereby preventing viral entry.

## 38.  B (MHC-I)

Virus-infected cells may show a reduction in the number of MHC-I molecules on their cell surface. The presence of MHC-I is recognised as 'self' by natural killer cells and Th1 cells. Therefore, a reduction in MHC-I can be identified as 'non-self', meaning that it can be destroyed by natural killer cells and T killer cells.

## 39.  A (*Klebsiella pneumoniae*)

The main infectious causes of cavitating lung lesions are *Streptococcus pneumoniae*, *Klebsiella pneumoniae*, *Staphylococcus aureus* and *Mycobacterium tuberculosis*. Furthermore, *Klebsiella* is a relatively common cause of pneumonia in patients with a history of alcohol excess. Other non-infectious causes of cavitating lung lesions include squamous cell lung cancer, rheumatoid arthritis and granulomatosis with polyangiitis.

*Haemophilus influenzae*, *Legionella pneumophila* and *Mycoplasma pneumoniae* are not classically associated with cavitating lung lesions. *Mycobacterium tuberculosis* can cause cavitating lung lesions, however, it is likely to present with a chronic history of weight loss, cough and general constitutional upset.

## 40.  B (Bacterial cell death)

A Jarisch–Herxheimer reaction is an overwhelming inflammatory reaction to bacterial endotoxins that are released from bacteria as they lyse due to antibiotic treatment. It can manifest similarly to sepsis and it can be life-threatening. It is classically associated with the treatment of syphilis but may also occur in the treatment of spirochete infections such as Lyme disease. It is usually treated with anti-inflammatory agents such as aspirin.

Serum sickness refers to a hypersensitivity reaction to antibodies from a non-human source (e.g. antivenom). It tends to occur 5–10 days after exposure and presents with a fever, rash and joint pain. Anaphylaxis is an IgE-mediated severe allergic reaction which is likely to occur within minutes of exposure to an allergen and will cause airway compromise (due to laryngeal oedema), urticaria and shock. Antibody-dependent enhancement refers to a phenomenon in which antibody binding enhances the virulence of a virus. It is most commonly associated with dengue virus. Inflammatory cell margination occurs in infection as cells arrest along the endothelial membrane prior to entering the diseased tissues, however, this would not be the main cause of this patient's worsening clinical state.

# Genetics

## Questions

1. A 6-year-old boy with a developmental abnormality is undergoing several genetic investigations. He is found to have an unbalanced chromosomal abnormality at 7q11.23.

   Which of the following features would be suggestive of Williams syndrome?

   A Long philtrum, broad nose, delayed speech
   B Abnormality of the aorta, flat eyebrows, delayed speech development
   C Long philtrum, upturned nose, friendly personality
   D Short philtrum, arched eyebrows, friendly personality
   E Abnormality of the aorta, flat eyebrows, impaired social interaction

2. What type of inheritance pattern is shown in this diagram?

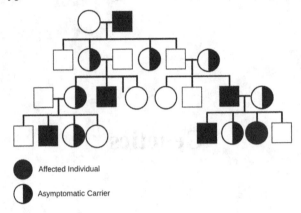

A Autosomal recessive
B Autosomal dominant
C X-linked recessive
D X-linked dominant
E Cannot be deduced

3. A 34-year-old pregnant woman is concerned about the risk of her newborn having Duchenne muscular dystrophy (X-linked recessive inheritance) as her father suffered from the disease. Her partner does not have the disease and is not a carrier.
Which of the following is the most appropriate next step for this patient?

A No further investigation necessary as there is no risk of inheritance
B Routine scan to check for skeletal dysplasia
C Amniocentesis
D Cell-free foetal DNA
E Chorionic villus sampling

4. A 33-year-old man has been referred to the gastroenterology department after developing features of chronic liver disease. He does not drink, and his hepatitis screen is clear. His haematinics reveal a very

high ferritin level and transferrin saturation, so a diagnosis of hereditary haemochromatosis is made. His close relatives were tested, and his mother is found to be homozygous for the hereditary haemochromatosis mutation. She has never been symptomatic.

Which of the following best explains the difference in presentation between the mother and son?

A A second gene modifying the phenotypic expression of C282Y
B Hereditary haemochromatosis is X-linked
C Differences in environmental factors change the disease phenotype
D Differential effects in males compared to females
E They have inherited different mutations of the C282Y gene

5. The Ras gene, once mutated and activated, leads to the development of cancer.
   Which of the following terms best describes the Ras gene?

   A Proto-oncogene
   B Oncogene
   C Tumour suppressor gene
   D Anti-apoptotic gene
   E Promoter gene

6. A 21-year-old man has asked to speak to a genetic counsellor. His father has Leber's Hereditary Optic Neuropathy (LHON), a disease caused by genetic mutations in mitochondrial DNA, which resulted in him losing his vision in his twenties. The patient's mother does not have LHON.
   What is the risk of this patient having LHON?

   A 0
   B 0.25
   C 0.5
   D 1
   E More information required

7. Fabry disease is a lysosomal storage disorder that is caused by a deficiency in alpha-galactosidase A. It results from a genetic defect that leads to misfolding of the enzyme.
   Which type of treatment would be most suitable for this type of genetic disease?

   A  Pharmacological receptor agonist
   B  In vivo gene therapy supplement
   C  Pharmacological chaperones
   D  Stop codon read through
   E  Combination therapy

8. Sickle cell disease arises due to a point mutation at codon 6 of the beta-globin gene. It arises from a change in an amino acid from glutamic acid to valine, which results in the haemoglobin having a tendency to precipitate under certain conditions.
   What type of mutation is implicated in sickle cell disease?

   A  Silent
   B  Missense
   C  Nonsense
   D  Frameshift
   E  Inversion

9. Two patients, a 21-year-old woman and a 14-year-old boy, are known to the cystic fibrosis clinic. They are both homozygous for a mutation in Delta F508, which impairs the production of the cystic fibrosis transmembrane conductance regulator. The 14-year-old patient, however, has considerably more severe disease with frequent admissions for severe respiratory tract infections.
   Which of the following best explains the difference in disease progression between these patients?

   A  The patients inherited different mutations of the same gene
   B  Presence of different gene modifiers altering the disease phenotype

    **C** Differential effects in males and females

    **D** Different numbers of trinucleotide repeats

    **E** Environmental factors

10. Which enzymes bind onto promoter regions to initiate transcription?

    **A** DNA helicase

    **B** DNA polymerase

    **C** RNA polymerase II

    **D** Aminoacyl-tRNA synthetase

    **E** Peptidyl transferase

11. A 28-year-old pregnant woman with a family history of haemophilia A attends the fertility clinic and is concerned about the risk of her child being affected by the disease.

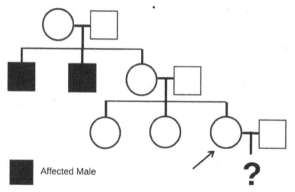

What is the risk of her child having haemophilia A?

    **A** 0

    **B** 1/8

    **C** 1/16

    **D** 1/64

    **E** 1/128

12. A 53-year-old man has been referred via the 2-week wait pathway with rectal bleeding. He is rather anxious as he has a family history

of gastrointestinal stromal tumours. A mass is identified on endoscopy and a biopsy is taken.

Which of the following is a proto-oncogene implicated in the development of gastrointestinal stromal tumours?

    A  KIT
    B  BRCA
    C  MENI
    D  TP53
    E  Rb

13. What type of chromosomal abnormality causes Klinefelter syndrome (XXY)?

    A  Isochromosomes
    B  Robertsonian translocation
    C  Duplications
    D  Pericentric inversions
    E  Nondisjunction

14. The coding strand of a specific gene begins as 5′ATGTGCGAA3′. What is the base sequence of the corresponding mRNA?

    A  5′AUGUGCGAA3′
    B  3′AUGUGCGAA5′
    C  3′UACACGCUU5′
    D  5′UACACGCUU3′
    E  3′TACACGCTT5′

15. Which molecule is downregulated within epithelial cells to enable cancer cell infiltration?

    A  E-selectin
    B  E-cadherin
    C  Fibronectin

**D** PSGL-I

**E** PECAM-I

16. A 43-year-old woman has become pregnant for the first time after several years of trying. She has read about the increased risk of Down syndrome in older mothers. She is currently at 14 weeks gestation and would like her baby to be screened for Down syndrome.

    Which of the following is the most appropriate initial screening tool for Down syndrome?

    **A** Routine ultrasound and blood test

    **B** Cell-free foetal DNA

    **C** Chorionic villus sampling

    **D** Amniocentesis

    **E** Maternal genome sequencing

17. A 49-year-old man has been referred to the neurology outpatient clinic with a new diagnosis of Huntington's disease. The symptoms are relatively mild at present; however, he is quite distressed by the diagnosis because he has seen how his mother had suffered with it. His mother started showing symptoms at the age of 65 years.

    Which of the following explains the difference in the age of onset between the mother and son?

    **A** Different environmental interactions that modify the disease phenotype

    **B** Son is homozygous whereas the mother is heterozygous

    **C** Different mutations in the same gene

    **D** Earlier age of onset in male patients

    **E** Son has greater number of trinucleotide repeats

18. A patient (indicated by the arrow below) attends the genetic counselling clinic as she is hoping to start a family with her partner. Both the patient and her partner have a family history of Tay Sachs disease.

The patient's father and the partner's mother have no family history of Tay Sachs and are not carriers.

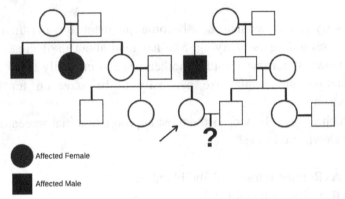

○ Affected Female

■ Affected Male

Based on the information above, what is the probability of the child being affected?

A  1/32
B  1/36
C  1/48
D  1/64
E  1/72

19. A 22-year-old woman attends a genetic counselling clinic to discuss her family history of X-linked agammaglobulinaemia. She explains that her maternal uncle and her brother have the disease and have suffered from recurrent infections throughout their lives. She has no past medical history of note.
    Based on the information provided, what is the probability of her being a carrier of the disease?

A  0%
B  25%
C  50%
D  75%
E  100%

20. A 3-day-old neonate has developed abdominal distension and vomiting. It is also noted that he has still not passed meconium and a diagnosis of Hirschsprung disease is suspected. It occurs due to the failure of craniocaudal migration of vagal neural crest cells within the colon.

Which cell lineage are these neural crest cells derived from?

    **A** Endoderm
    **B** Ectoderm
    **C** Mesoderm
    **D** Epiblast
    **E** Hypoblast

## Answers

### 1.  C (Long philtrum, upturned nose, friendly personality)

Williams syndrome is caused by a 7q11.23 deletion. It manifests with morphological abnormalities such as a long philtrum, short, upturned nose and arched eyebrows. Patients with Williams syndrome are also classically described as having a friendly personality. 7q11.23 duplication syndrome is a condition that results from an abnormality in the same gene. It typically manifests with a short philtrum, broad nose and flat eyebrows. Abnormalities of the aorta are seen in both Williams syndrome (supravalvular aortic stenosis) and 7q11.23 deletion (aortic dilatation). Behaviourally, patients with 7q11.23 duplication demonstrate features of autism such as impaired social interaction.

### 2.  C (X-linked recessive)

In this example, primarily males are affected and there is no vertical transmission of the disease between males. Furthermore, all daughters of affected males are carriers thus suggestive of an X-linked recessive pattern of inheritance.

### 3.  B (Routine scan to check for skeletal dysplasia)

Routine scans looking at nuchal thickness are conducted between 10–14 weeks gestation. These scans are useful for determining the risk of an unborn child developing various chromosomal abnormalities (e.g. Down syndrome) and skeletal dysplasias. In this case, the patient's father had Duchenne muscular dystrophy, which, given that it is X-linked recessive, would mean that she is a carrier. Therefore, even though her partner does not carry the gene, the child has a 50% risk of having the disease if it is a boy.

### 4.  D (Differential effects in males compared to females)

Hereditary haemochromatosis is an autosomal recessive disorder caused by a mutation in the HFE gene which encodes hepcidin — a protein that regulates iron absorption. Dysfunction of hepcidin results in excess iron absorption from the gastrointestinal tract. The iron can deposit in various organs across the body resulting in a number of clinical manifestations, including cirrhosis, heart failure and diabetes mellitus. Females tend to be relatively protected from the effects of hereditary haemochromatosis as they naturally have a lower haemoglobin concentration and menstrual bleeding regularly reduces their total body iron content.

## 5. A (Proto-oncogene)

A proto-oncogene is a normal gene that has some sort of normal cellular function. Once mutated, however, they become oncogenes that promote disordered cell proliferation and the development of cancer. Tumour suppressor genes prevent aberrant cell division. The disabling of tumour suppressor genes increases the risk of developing cancer.

## 6. A (0)

Leber's hereditary optic neuropathy (LHON) is an example of a mitochondrial disorder. Mitochondria is strictly maternally inherited — i.e. our mitochondria have come from our mother. Therefore, mitochondrial disorders can only be inherited from mother to child. Another example of mitochondrial disorder is MELAS (mitochondrial encephalopathy, lactic acidosis and stroke-like symptoms). In this case, the patient's mother does not have LHON, so he is not at risk of having LHON.

## 7. C (Pharmacological chaperones)

Protein folding occurs within the endoplasmic reticulum and is regulated by chaperone proteins. Molecular chaperones in the endoplasmic reticulum are designated to support nascent proteins entering the endoplasmic reticulum and facilitate their folding into the correct conformation. In this particular example of Fabry disease, Migalastat is a pharmacological chaperone that works by binding to the active site of the misfolded alpha-galactosidase A and helps it change into the correct, functional conformation.

A pharmacological receptor agonist is an agent that activates a receptor thereby causing a downstream cellular effect. Salbutamol is an example of a receptor agonist as it stimulates $\beta_2$ adrenergic receptors. In vivo gene therapy supplementation involves using viral vectors to deliver genes that are defective or absent in certain disease states. Nonsense mutations are caused by premature stop codons within the mRNA sequence. Stop codons cease ribosomal translation of the protein, thereby creating a truncated and dysfunctional protein. Stop codon readthrough involves the binding of a nonsense suppressor which prevents premature truncation of the protein. Ataluren is a drug used in the treatment of Duchenne muscular dystrophy. It inhibits premature stop codons thereby allowing the formation of functional dystrophin. Combination therapy involves a combination of chaperon and activator molecules that support the functional activity of a misfolded cell-surface protein. Ivacaftor/Lumacaftor is a combination drug used in the treatment of cystic fibrosis that works by increasing channel opening and enhances trafficking of the protein to the cell surface.

### 8.  B (Missense)

A missense mutation is a point mutation that results in a change in a single amino acid within the polypeptide sequence. In the case of sickle cell disease, the mutation results in a change in the amino acid from glutamic acid to valine. This results in the formation of abnormal haemoglobin S (HbS) which has a tendency to polymerise in certain environments (e.g. hypoxia) and change the morphology of a red cell into a sickle shape.

A silent mutation is when a change in the nuclear code does not result in any change in the amino acid sequence produced. This is because multiple trinucleotide base sequences can encode the same amino acid. A nonsense mutation is when a mutation changes a codon that previously encoded an amino acid into a stop codon. This will terminate the polypeptide chain prematurely, resulting in the formation of a defective protein. Frameshift mutations occur due to base deletions and insertions that offset the reading frame during translation. This means that the codons are read entirely differently such that a completely different polypeptide is produced. An inversion is when a segment of a chromosome is reversed end to end.

## 9. B (Presence of different gene modifiers altering the disease phenotype)

Gene modifiers are genes that can affect the expression of the disease-causing gene, thereby affecting disease phenotype. The TGFB-1 gene is one such example that is associated with severe lung disease in patients with cystic fibrosis. Another example is the FCGR2A gene which increases the risk of developing chronic *Pseudomonas* infection in cystic fibrosis.

## 10. C (RNA polymerase II)

Transcription is the process by which mRNA (transcript) is produced, which is then translated into a specific polypeptide sequence. A promoter region is a sequence of non-coding nucleotides (e.g. TATA box) that is located upstream of the segment that needs to be transcribed. RNA polymerase II binds onto the TATA box which allows the process of transcription to begin. This works by separating the two strands of the DNA thereby exposing the template strand for the binding of RNA nucleotides. RNA polymerase then catalyses the formation of phosphodiester bonds between adjacent RNA nucleotides, resulting in the formation of a strand of mRNA.

DNA helicase separates the template and coding strands of DNA during DNA replication. DNA polymerase catalyses the formation of phosphodiester bonds between adjacent DNA nucleotides in DNA replication. Aminoacyl-tRNA synthetase facilitates the matching of each amino acid to the appropriate RNA codon during translation. Peptidyl transferase is responsible for forming peptide bonds between adjacent amino acids during translation.

## 11. C (1/16)

Haemophilia A is an X-linked recessive condition that predominantly affects males. In this case, the female in generation I is a carrier as she has two affected sons. This means that the female in generation II has a ½ chance of being a carrier. As her daughter (patient in this case) will inherit one of her two X chromosomes, the patient will have a ¼ chance of being a carrier (½ × ½). If we assume that the patient is a carrier, then the possible genotypes of her child are shown by the following Punnett square.

Haemophilia A = h

|      | Xh                   | XH    |
|------|----------------------|-------|
| XH   | XH Xh                | XH XH |
| Y    | Xh Y (Affected male) | XH Y  |

This shows that there is a ¼ chance of having an affected child if the patient is a carrier. Therefore, to figure out the overall probability of this patient having a child with haemophilia A, it would be ¼ × ¼ = 1/16.

## 12. A (KIT)

Proto-oncogenes are genes that have a normal cellular function involving cell division. However, a gain of function mutation can result in the formation of an oncogene which promotes unregulated cell division and the development of cancer. The KIT proto-oncogene encodes a tyrosine kinase receptor. Once mutated, it can result in the constant activation of this receptor which results in excessive intracellular signalling and growth factor expression. This, ultimately, results in uncontrolled cell division.

BRCA, MEN1, TP53 and Rb are tumour suppressor genes. They are genes that regulate cell division and loss of function of these genes can result in an increased risk of aberrant cell signalling and excessive cell proliferation.

## 13. E (Nondisjunction)

A chromosome nondisjunction occurs when a pair of sister chromatids fail to separate during meiosis. This results in an abnormal number of chromosomes in the daughter cells (in this case, gametes). In Klinefelter syndrome, a single gamete inherits two copies of the X chromosome from the mother, which means that, during fusion, the zygote produced will have three sex chromosomes (XXY). This gives an overall karyotype of 47 XXY.

An isochromosome is a type of chromosomal abnormality in which the arms of the chromosomes are mirror images of each other. This is due to an aberrant split of the chromosomes at the chromatid which results in the formation of one chromosome composed of just the short arms and one chromosome composed of just the long arms. A Robertsonian translocation is a chromosomal abnormality that occurs between two acrocentric chromosomes in which a chromosome is formed by the parts of two chromosomes (e.g. 13 and 14). A translocation carrier will be asymptomatic, however, during fertilisation, it can result in the formation of a zygote with an extra copy of a chromosome. A duplication occurs when part of a chromosomal segment is duplicated. A pericentric inversion is when a segment of chromosome is inverted around the centromere.

## 14. A (5′AUGUGCGAA3′)

During transcription mRNA is formed by the binding of RNA nucleotides to the template (antisense) DNA strand in a 5′ to 3′ direction. The phosphodiester bonds are formed by the action of RNA polymerase. In this case, the code provided is the coding strand. Therefore, the RNA will be generated from the opposing (antisense) strand. The RNA strand should, thus, be identical to the coding strand except for the use of uracil instead of thymine.

## 15. B (E-cadherin)

E-cadherin is a cell-to-cell adhesion molecule that forms adherens junctions between adjacent epithelial cells. This maintains epithelial integrity. The downregulation of E-cadherins compromises the integrity of the epithelium and increases the risk of infiltration by tumour cells. Once malignant cells have breached the basement membrane, they can spread via the lymphatics and circulation.

E-selectins are cell surface adhesion proteins expressed by endothelial cells which mediate the attachment of leukocytes to the endothelial surface. Fibronectin is a multi-adhesive glycoprotein supporting cell adhesion within the basement membrane. PSGL-I is an adhesion molecule expressed by neutrophils and T-cells during chemotaxis. Platelet endothelial cell adhesion molecule mediates the rearrangement of the neutrophil cytoskeleton thereby facilitating neutrophil transmigration.

### 16. A (Routine ultrasound and blood test)

A routine scan with blood tests is offered at 10–14 weeks' gestation for all women. The scan looks at the nuchal translucency and the blood tests measure $\beta$-hCG and PAPP-A. The results of these tests are amalgamated to form the 'combined test' which can identify pregnancies that are at high risk of Down, Patau, Edwards' and Turner syndrome.

Cell free-foetal DNA is a non-invasive prenatal diagnostic technique that works by analysing the foetal DNA fragments that can be found in the maternal circulation during pregnancy. Chorionic villus sampling involves taking a transabdominal or transvaginal sample of the chorionic villi of the placenta. This will contain some foetal DNA that can be analysed for various genetic abnormalities such as Down syndrome. Amniocentesis is a technique by which a sample of amniotic fluid is taken for analysis. It will contain some foetal DNA which can be analysed for chromosomal abnormalities. Down syndrome is an aneuploidy not an inherited condition, so genome sequencing will be of no benefit.

### 17. E (Son has greater number of trinucleotide repeats)

Huntington's disease is an autosomal dominant genetic disorder resulting from the degeneration of GABAergic neurones in the striatum, caudate and putamen. It results in progressively worsening chorea. It is caused by a CAG trinucleotide repeat in the Huntingtin gene. The number of CAG repeats increases as the disease passes down generations and this results in an earlier age of onset of the disease — a phenomenon known as anticipation.

## 18. B (1/36)

Tay–Sachs disease is an autosomal recessive disorder that results in degeneration of neurones within the central nervous system. Its inheritance pattern can be deduced from the pedigree as two unaffected parents give rise to affected children.

In the first generation on both sides, the genotypes of both parents are Xx (x being the recessive allele) as they have a child or children affected by the disease but they, themselves, are unaffected. Therefore, the risk of the patient's mother and the partner's father being a carrier can be expressed in the Punnett square below. The homozygous recessive genotype (xx) can be discounted as it would have appeared on the pedigree. Therefore, there are three possible genotypes for the individuals in the second generation and the probability of being a carrier is ⅔.

|   | X | x |
|---|---|---|
| X | XX | Xx (Carrier) |
| x | Xx (Carrier) | xx (Affected) |

In the second generation, we know that the patient's father and the partner's mother are not carriers so, assuming that their other parent was a carrier, their risk of being a carrier is ½ (see below).

|   | X | X |
|---|---|---|
| X | XX | XX |
| x | Xx (Carrier) | Xx (Carrier) |

We then multiply the probability of the parent in the second generation being a carrier (⅔) with the probability of the patient and her partner being a carrier assuming that their parent is a carrier (½). This gives a ⅓ risk of being a carrier for both the patient and her partner as their inheritance follows similar generational patterns.

The risk of two carriers having an affected individual is ¼ (see next page).

|   | X | x |
|---|---|---|
| X | XX | Xx (Carrier) |
| x | Xx (Carrier) | xx **(Affected)** |

Therefore, the probability of the child being affected is equal to the chance of their mother being a carrier (⅓) multiplied by the chance of their father being a carrier (⅓) multiplied by the chance of two carriers having an affected child (¼). This gives an overall risk of 1/36.

## 19. C (50%)

X-linked agammaglobulinaemia is an X-linked recessive disorder that is characterised by an inability to produce plasma cells and, therefore, an inability to produce antibodies. This leads to an increased risk of infections, especially by encapsulated organisms such as *Streptococcus pneumoniae*. The mainstay of treatment is regular IV immunoglobulin to provide patients with a degree of passive immunity.

As this patient's brother has the disease, it can be assumed that their mother is a carrier. As she will only inherit one of her mother's two X chromosomes, there is a 50% chance that she will be a carrier. There is no mention of her father having the disease, so it can be assumed that he has a normal X chromosome.

## 20. B (Ectoderm)

During early embryological development, three germ layers form: endoderm, ectoderm and mesoderm. The ectoderm is the outermost layer of embryonic cells and it gives rise to neural crest cells and epithelial tissues. Some neural crest cells will migrate in craniocaudal direction and begin to form the enteric nervous system. The failure of this migration can result in the absence of enteric ganglion cells in the distal portion of the gastrointestinal tract which, in turn, leads to the failure of peristaltic movements and, hence, constipation. The treatment of Hirschsprung disease involves surgically excising the affected portion of the bowel.

# Mock Exam

## Questions

1. Peyer's patches are a form of gut-associated lymphoid tissue which contains a B-cell zone where dendritic cells present antigens to B-cells, resulting in antibody class switching.
   Which antibodies are secreted by activated B-cells in Peyer's patches?

   A  IgA
   B  IgM
   C  IgG
   D  IgE
   E  IgD

2. A 61-year-old man has been admitted to the infectious diseases ward after developing COVID-19 pneumonitis. He had desaturated to 88% on admission, so has been started on oxygen therapy and dexamethasone. A set of blood is taken on the second day of his admission.
   Which of the following changes is likely to be seen on this blood test compared to his first blood test upon admission?

   A  Decreased lymphocytes
   B  Decreased albumin

    C  Increased neutrophils
    D  Increased CRP
    E  Increased platelets

3. A 45-year-old man has been admitted to the general medical ward after being diagnosed with a pulmonary embolism. He begins treatment with low molecular weight heparin; however, he is morbidly obese, so ongoing anticoagulation with warfarin is recommended as he will require regular monitoring. He is started on warfarin treatment; however, he will need to remain on low molecular weight heparin until his INR is maintained within the therapeutic range. Warfarin is known to cause an initial prothrombotic phase.
Inhibition of which of the following clotting factors is responsible for this effect?

    A  Antithrombin III
    B  Thrombomodulin
    C  Protein C
    D  Plasmin
    E  Thrombin

4. Cystic fibrosis is a condition in which patients produce viscous secretions within their respiratory, gastrointestinal and urogenital tract, resulting in a number of complications such as respiratory tract infections and infertility. It is caused by a mutation in the cystic fibrosis transmembrane conductance regulator, which is a chloride channel.
Which of the following is the first investigation used to screen for cystic fibrosis in a newborn?

    A  Immunoreactive trypsinogen
    B  Delta F508 test
    C  Sweat test
    D  Genome sequencing
    E  Sputum osmolality

5. A 55-year-old man with a background of Crohn's disease has been noted to have become increasingly fluid overloaded after being admitted with a flare. A urine dipstick reveals a markedly elevated level of protein and renal amyloidosis is suspected. A renal biopsy is requested to confirm the diagnosis.
   Which of the following stains would be most appropriate in this instance?

   A  Ziehl–Neelsen
   B  Congo Red
   C  Auramine
   D  India Ink
   E  Sudan Black

6. A 66-year-old man who has been admitted to hospital with an infective exacerbation of COPD has been treated with high flow oxygen. He remained on 15 L/min of oxygen via a non-rebreather mask despite an improvement in his oxygen saturation. The patient is noted to have become drowsy on the second day of his admission, and an ABG reveals a high $PaO_2$ and a high $PaCO_2$.
   Which of the following describes the effect of oxygen on the binding of carbon dioxide to haemoglobin?

   A  Bohr effect
   B  Venturi effect
   C  Bernoulli principle
   D  Haldane effect
   E  Boyle's law

7. A 56-year-old woman has recently been diagnosed with rheumatoid arthritis after complaining of bilateral swelling and pain in her fingers over the preceding 6 months. Rheumatoid arthritis is driven by excessive release of proinflammatory cytokines such as TNF-$\alpha$ and IL1. Which of the following cells is primarily responsible for the release of these cytokines in rheumatoid arthritis?

    **A** Neutrophils
    **B** CD8+ T lymphocytes
    **C** Th17 lymphocytes
    **D** Macrophages
    **E** Eosinophils

8. A 41-year-old woman has attended a clinic appointment to review the management of her coeliac disease. Ahead of the appointment she has a blood test, and the blood film report mentions the presence of Howell–Jolly bodies.
   Which complication of coeliac disease is this suggestive of?

    **A** Enteropathy-associated T-cell lymphoma
    **B** Hyposplenism
    **C** Bone marrow failure
    **D** Vitamin B12 deficiency
    **E** Iron deficiency

9. A 5-year-old boy is currently being investigated in the developmental paediatrics clinic after concerns about his eating habits and large body habitus. Since a very young age, he has had an insatiable appetite and has remained consistently on the 99th centile for weight.
   A defect in which of the following chromosomes could explain his condition?

    **A** Maternal chromosome 6
    **B** Paternal chromosome 6
    **C** Maternal chromosome 15
    **D** Paternal chromosome 15
    **E** Maternal chromosome 13

10. Carmustine is a chemotherapy drug that is used to treat Hodgkin lymphoma by inhibiting DNA synthesis and RNA translation.
    During which state of the cell cycle does Carmustine act?

**A** G1
**B** G2
**C** S phase
**D** Mitosis
**E** Cytokinesis

11. A 26-year-old man has been admitted under the surgical team after presenting with acute abdominal pain. An ultrasound scan reveals a dilated appendix suggestive of acute appendicitis. A panel of blood tests is requested prior to his laparoscopic appendicectomy (results below).

Hb: 92 g/L (130–170)
MCV: 68 fL (82–100)
WCC: $19.5 \times 10^9$/L (4–11)
Neut: $16.2 \times 10^9$/L (2–7)
CRP: 351 mg/L (< 0.6)
Iron: 16 $\mu$mol/L (10–30)

He has no past medical history, but he mentions that both his parents have been found to be anaemic in the past.
Which of the following additional blood test parameters would be useful in establishing a diagnosis?

**A** Ferritin
**B** HbA2
**C** Vitamin B12
**D** Direct antiglobulin test
**E** Lymphoblast count

12. A 3-year-old boy has been urgently referred to the paediatric outpatient clinic after his GP noted faltering growth on his charts. Over the past 8 months, he has developed five chest infections, two of which had required hospital admission. On examination, he appears small for his age and is notably pale with bruising across his arms and legs.

Based on the information provided, what is the most likely diagnosis?

   **A** Acute myeloid leukaemia
   **B** Acute lymphoblastic leukaemia
   **C** Chronic myeloid leukaemia
   **D** Chronic lymphocytic leukaemia
   **E** Hodgkin lymphoma

13. Gastrointestinal bacterial growth is limited by the presence of gut enzymes.
    Which region of the gastrointestinal tract is most heavily colonised by bacteria?

   **A** Stomach
   **B** Duodenum
   **C** Jejunum
   **D** Ileum
   **E** Colon

14. Which genetic disorder is most likely to cause the inheritance pattern shown in this pedigree?

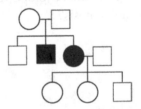

   **A** Duchenne muscular dystrophy
   **B** Huntington disease
   **C** Phenylketonuria
   **D** Marfan syndrome
   **E** Fragile X syndrome

15. A 22-year-old man, who has recently been diagnosed with Crohn's disease, has been started on azathioprine to try and reduce the frequency and severity of his exacerbations.

Which of the following is a major adverse effect of azathioprine?

A Diarrhoea
B Bone marrow suppression
C Secondary polycythaemia
D Acute kidney injury
E Transient neutrophilia

16. A 55-year-old man, with a background of G6PD deficiency, has been admitted to the hospital with a chest infection. His admission blood test results are shown below.

Hb: 62 g/L (130–170)
MCV: 108 fL (82–100)
WCC: 16.1 × 10^9/L (4–11)
Neut: 12.5 × 10^9/L (2–7)
CRP: 129 mg/L (<0.6)

Which of the following additional blood test markers would you expect to be low in this case?

A Lactate dehydrogenase
B Bilirubin
C Haptoglobin
D Reticulocytes
E Platelets

17. Two identical twins have been diagnosed with multiple endocrine neoplasia type I upon genetic testing — an autosomal dominant disease that is associated with pituitary adenomas, parathyroid adenomas and neuroendocrine tumours of the gastrointestinal tract. One twin has severe symptoms associated with the endocrine complications of the disease, whilst the other is asymptomatic.
What is the most likely cause of the difference in their phenotypes?

A They have inherited different mutations of the same gene
B They have inherited the same mutation from different parental chromosomes

    **C** A second gene is modifying the disease phenotype

    **D** Differences in environmental factors

    **E** Different effects in males and females

18. Which of the following can cause an increase in serum lactate concentration?

    **A** Salbutamol

    **B** Hypertension

    **C** Dialysis

    **D** Hyperglycaemia

    **E** Oxygen therapy

19. A 66-year-old man with a background of COPD, end-stage renal failure and hypertension, has been admitted to the acute medical unit after presenting with a cough and a fever. He is currently receiving antibiotics to cover a chest infection. As part of his admission work-up, he has an ECG, which reveals normal sinus rhythm and a blood test (see below).

    Na: 141 mmol/L (135–145)

    K: 4.6 mmol/L (3.5–5.5)

    Ur: 5.4 mmol/L (<7)

    Creat: 512 µmol/L (<90)

    Troponin (0 hr): 155 ng/L (<14)

    Troponin (3 hr): 143 ng/L (<14)

    Which of the following is most likely to have caused a rise in his troponin?

    **A** Pulmonary embolism

    **B** Myocardial infarction

    **C** Unstable angina

    **D** Renal failure

    **E** Exacerbation of asthma

20. A 32-year-old woman presents to her GP with a long history of a non-productive cough, shortness of breath and painful knees. She is referred to the respiratory outpatient clinic and has a chest X-ray which reveals bilateral hilar lymphadenopathy. Furthermore, a blood test reveals mild hypercalcaemia.

Given the most likely diagnosis, which of the following cell types is responsible for the high calcium concentration seen in this disease?

    **A** Neutrophils
    **B** Macrophages
    **C** Eosinophils
    **D** Basophils
    **E** T lymphocytes

# Answers

## 1. A (IgA)

Peyer's patches are a form of gut-associated lymphoid tissue (GALT) that are found within the small bowel, in particular the ileum. GALT have an important role in regulating the adaptive and innate immune systems. Epithelial dendritic cells will sample antigens within the epithelium. These antigens are then internalised and processed before being loaded onto MHC-II molecules and presented to naive B-cells within the lymphoid tissue. The interaction between antigen-presenting cells and B-cells results in antibody class-switching from IgM to IgA. The plasma cells will then secrete dimeric IgA, which binds to poly-Ig receptors on the basal surface of epithelial cells, and are internalised and processed within the cells before being secreted as secretory IgA into the intestinal lumen. Within the lumen, IgA will bind to antigens and prevent pathogen adhesion and entry.

## 2.  C (Increased neutrophils)

The administration of corticosteroids causes a transient neutrophilia as steroids reduce the expression of L-selectins within neutrophils, which are normally responsible for neutrophil adhesion to the surface of blood vessels. Reduced expression of these proteins will result in demargination of the neutrophils and, hence, increases the neutrophil count on blood tests.

Prolonged exposure to corticosteroids can have immunosuppressive effects resulting in a low lymphocyte count. Furthermore, many patients with COVID-19 will be lymphopenic. A decrease in albumin is often seen in acutely unwell patients. It is a negative acute phase protein. C-reactive protein is produced by the liver and acts as an opsonin that facilitates phagocytosis by macrophages. It is used as a nonspecific marker of infection and inflammation. A rise in platelet count is often seen in acute infectious and inflammatory conditions. It is a positive acute phase marker.

### 3. C (Protein C)

Warfarin is a vitamin K epoxide reductase inhibitor that causes anticoagulation by inhibiting the gamma-carboxylation of factors II, VII, IX and X. Warfarin also inhibits protein C and protein S which normally inactivate factor Va and factor VIIIa, thereby acting as part of the body's endogenous anticoagulant mechanism. The half-lives of protein C and protein S are shorter than the half-lives of the other clotting factors inhibited by warfarin, which means that, during the initial phase of warfarin treatment, protein C and S will be inhibited with no inhibition of the other clotting factors. This increases the risk of thrombus formation and, hence, requires additional anticoagulation with an alternative agent such as low molecular weight heparin.

### 4. A (Immunoreactive trypsinogen)

Cystic fibrosis is usually diagnosed during newborn screening. All newborns in the UK will have a heel prick test which samples a small amount of blood for a panel of tests that screen for various inherited conditions such as cystic fibrosis, sickle cell disease, hypothyroidism and phenylketonuria. Immunoreactive trypsinogen (IRT) is a pancreatic enzyme that is elevated in patients with cystic fibrosis. Patients with levels of IRT that are above the 99.5th centile will be tested for the four most common mutations that cause cystic fibrosis. The newborn will then go on to have a sweat test which looks at the sodium concentration of the sweat (increased in cystic fibrosis).

### 5. B (Congo Red)

Congo Red stain is used to identify amyloid deposits within the kidneys. Amyloidosis is a condition in which abnormal amyloid proteins accumulate in various tissues across the body (most notably the kidneys, resulting in nephrotic syndrome). It can occur as a consequence of chronic inflammatory conditions (such as Crohn's disease), which are associated with a persistently elevated level of the acute phase protein, serum amyloid A. It can also occur due to the aggregation of immunoglobulin light chains in multiple myeloma. The visualisation of apple-green birefrin-gence on a renal biopsy stained with Congo Red is suggestive of renal amyloidosis.

Ziehl–Neelsen and Auramine stains are used in the identification of *Mycobacterium tuberculosis*. India Ink is used in the identification of *Cryptococcus neoformans*. Prussian Blue is used to identify iron deposi-tion within tissues.

### 6.  D (Haldane effect)

The Haldane effect describes the relationship between the partial pressure of oxygen and the affinity of haemoglobin for carbon dioxide. Carbon dioxide is acidic, so the accumulation of carbon dioxide within the blood due to respiratory issues can result in respiratory acidosis. Haemoglobin is one of the body's mechanisms of buffering carbon dioxide and prevent-ing acidosis. The absorption of high concentrations of oxygen into the circulation decreases the affinity of haemoglobin for carbon dioxide, thereby resulting in an increase in arterial carbon dioxide concentration. The carbon dioxide will then react with water and be converted to car-bonic acid which, subsequently, will dissociate into protons (causing aci-dosis) and bicarbonate. This is one of the mechanisms by which hyperoxygenation of patients with chronic carbon dioxide retention can lead to worsening hypercapnia.

The Bohr effect describes the effect of carbon dioxide concentration on the affinity of haemoglobin for oxygen. In the presence of high concentra-tions of carbon dioxide, the affinity of haemoglobin for oxygen will increase. The Venturi effect is a principle of physics that states that when a fluid or gas passes through a narrowing, the pressure exerted within that narrowing will decrease. This is one of the principles upon which the design of the Venturi mask is based. The Bernoulli principle states that the passage of a fluid or gas through a narrowing will result in an increase in the speed of the fluid or gas. Boyle's law states that the pressure exerted by a given mass of a gas at a constant temperature is inversely propor-tional to the volume it occupies.

## 7. D (Macrophages)

Rheumatoid arthritis is a systemic inflammatory condition that primarily affects the small joints of the hands and feet. It is thought to occur due to the citrullination of peptides within the synovium which enables them to be recognised as foreign by the immune system (with subsequent generation of anti-cyclic citrullinated peptide antibodies). The antibodies can activate macrophages which then release various proinflammatory cytokines such as TNF-$\alpha$ and IL1. This can then result in increased expression of matrix metalloproteinases which contribute to joint destruction.

## 8. B (Hyposplenism)

Hyposplenism is a known complication of coeliac disease. The spleen is the site of breakdown of red cells, so hyposplenism can result in a number of blood film changes such as Howell–Jolly bodies (aggregates of DNA), target cells and acanthocytes. Other complications of coeliac disease include vitamin B12 and folic acid deficiency (causing megaloblastic anaemia) and iron deficiency (causing microcytic anaemia).

## 9. D (Paternal chromosome 15)

Genomic imprinting is a phenomenon in which the expression of genetic material depends on whether it has been inherited from the mother or the father. Prader-Willi syndrome is an example of an imprinting disorder which is caused by the inheritance of a defective copy of the paternal chromosome 15. It is characterised by an insatiable appetite which results in obesity and type II diabetes mellitus. Angelman syndrome is a related condition that is caused by inheritance of a defective copy of maternal chromosome 15. Features of Angelman syndrome include microcephaly, developmental disability and seizures.

## 10. C (S phase)

Semi-conservative DNA replication occurs during the synthesis phase of the cell cycle. During this phase, new histones are synthesised and bind with replicated DNA within the nucleus. Carmustine is a chemotherapy agent that forms crosslinks between DNA strands, thereby inhibiting DNA synthesis which, in turn, results in apoptosis.

During G1, the chromosomes form long, uncondensed threads that are wound around histone proteins. The cell is highly metabolically active during this stage and genes are being transcribed into mRNA molecules ahead of translation. During G2, the replicated DNA is checked for errors and corrected accordingly by DNA repair enzymes. Centrioles duplicate and migrate to opposite poles from which spindle fibres are formed. The chromosome condenses and prepares for mitosis. Mitosis (nuclear division) occurs during the M phase. Cytokinesis (cell division) also occurs during the M phase.

## 11. B (HbA2)

Thalassemia is a hereditary disorder of globin production that causes microcytic anaemia. Four globin chains combine with haem molecules to form haemoglobin. There are four types of globin: alpha, beta, gamma and delta. The majority of adult haemoglobin is HbA, which consists of two alpha chains and two beta chains. Beta thalassemia is a relatively common inherited condition in which patients produce reduced quantities of beta-globin. In response to this, the body will produce greater amounts of HbA2 — a variant form of adult haemoglobin which is made up of two alpha and two delta globin chains. It normally makes up a relatively small percentage of adult haemoglobin; however, in patients with thalassemia, the percentage of HbA2 will be markedly increased.

## 12. B (Acute lymphoblastic leukaemia)

Acute lymphoblastic leukaemia is the most common type of leukaemia in children. It is characterised by the production of excessive quantities of abnormal lymphoblasts within the bone marrow. The bone marrow becomes infiltrated by abnormal lymphoblasts thereby reducing its ability to produce normal, functional blood cells. This, consequently, leads to anaemia (reduced red cell production), easy bruising (reduced platelet production) and recurrent infections (reduced white cell production). Abnormal lymphoblasts will be detectable on a peripheral blood film and a bone marrow biopsy will confirm the diagnosis. Treatment may involve chemotherapy, radiotherapy and stem cell transplantation.

Acute myeloid leukaemia is more common in adults. Chronic myeloid leukaemia and chronic lymphocytic leukaemia may present with a slower onset of symptoms and it is more common in adults. Hodgkin lymphoma usually presents with lymphadenopathy and vague constitutional symptoms such as fever, weight loss and night sweats.

### 13. E (Colon)

The gut microbiome is a community of commensal organisms that are found within the gastrointestinal tract. There are four main groups of commensal organisms: bacteroidetes, firmicutes, actinobacteria and proteobacteria. The gut microbiome is carefully regulated by the ingestion and secretion of nutrients by the host, and the release of antimicrobial factors. The colon has a much greater population of microorganisms than the rest of the gastrointestinal tract.

### 14. C (Phenylketonuria)

Phenylketonuria is an autosomal recessive inborn error of amino acid metabolism that is characterised by a deficiency of phenylalanine hydroxylase. This results in elevated levels of phenylalanine that can cause abnormal myelination and neurotransmitter deficiency within the brain. Phenylketonuria is usually diagnosed during newborn screening and can be relatively easily treated by maintaining a low-protein diet. The pedigree in this image shows that unaffected couples can have affected children, and that both male and female children can be affected. This is suggestive of an autosomal recessive pattern of inheritance.

Duchenne muscular dystrophy is an X-linked recessive disorder. Huntington disease and Marfan syndrome are autosomal dominant disorders. Fragile X Syndrome is an X-linked dominant disorder.

### 15. B (Bone marrow suppression)

Azathioprine is an immunosuppressive medication that is used to treat inflammatory bowel disease and rheumatoid arthritis. Azathioprine is a prodrug that gets converted to 6-mercaptopurine. This is a purine analogue that gets incorporated into newly synthesised DNA and halts DNA replication. As it interferes with DNA replication, it can cause excessive bone marrow suppression and must be monitored closely. Thiopurine S-methyltransferase is an enzyme that is involved in the breakdown of azathioprine and reduced activity of this enzyme can increase the risk of bone marrow suppression in patients receiving azathioprine. Furthermore, xanthine oxidase is another enzyme that is involved in azathioprine metabolism so allopurinol (xanthine oxidase inhibitor used in the treatment of gout) should be avoided in patients receiving azathioprine.

### 16. C (Haptoglobin)

Haptoglobin is a protein produced by the liver that binds to free haemoglobin (released during haemolysis) and facilitates its removal via the spleen. Given its function in soaking up free haemoglobin, a decrease in haptoglobin concentration is seen in haemolytic conditions.

Lactate dehydrogenase is an intracellular enzyme that is found in most cells. A rise in lactate dehydrogenase is seen in any condition that causes cell death. Bilirubin is a by-product of red cell breakdown. Haemolysis is a cause of pre-hepatic jaundice. Reticulocytes are immature red cells that are released from the bone marrow in response to increased demand. Reticulocytes will rise in haemolytic anaemia. A change in platelet count is not usually associated with haemolytic anaemia.

### 17. D (Differences in environmental factors)

Phenotypic variability can result from genetic and environmental factors. As these patients are identical twins, they have the same genetic material and, hence, the same mutations. Therefore, the only variable that could account for a difference in their phenotype is their environment.

Many diseases with a genetic basis have been shown to have environmental triggers that can precipitate the onset of symptoms.

## 18. A (Salbutamol)

Lactic acid is a metabolic acid that is often measured in the evaluation of unwell patients. It is produced from pyruvate under anaerobic conditions. It is, therefore, used as a marker of tissue hypoxia (e.g. due to tissue hypoperfusion in sepsis). Another, less well acknowledged cause of lactic acidosis is increased glycolysis. As glucose, pyruvate and lactic acid exist in an equilibrium, anything that causes an increase in glucose entry into the cell and an increase in its conversion to pyruvate will, in turn, cause an increase in lactic acid. Adrenergic receptor stimulation can increase the rate of glycolysis within cells and, hence, increase the production of pyruvate from glucose, thereby increasing the production of lactate via anaerobic respiration. Salbutamol is a beta-adrenergic receptor agonist that can cause lactic acidosis through this mechanism.

## 19. D (Renal failure)

Troponins are proteins that are involved in muscle contraction. Troponin isoforms I and T are found mainly within the heart muscle and are often used as markers of myocardial injury (e.g. due to myocardial infarction). It is important to remember, however, that there are other factors that can result in a raised troponin. For example, troponins are primarily excreted via the kidneys so a severe impairment of renal function (as seen in this case) can result in a high serum troponin concentration in the absence of myocardial injury. As this patient has no ECG changes and no chest pain, his high troponin is unlikely to be caused by myocardial infarction. Furthermore, you would expect to see a rise in serial troponins taken after the onset of a myocardial infarction.

## 20. B (Macrophages)

Sarcoidosis is a systemic granulomatous condition of unknown aetiology that primarily affects the lungs but can also affect the joints and skin. It is characterised by the formation of non-caseating granulomas which are accumulations of macrophages and lymphocytes. In inflammatory states, the macrophages within the granuloma can express 1α-hydroxylase, which is a crucial enzyme in the activation of vitamin D. The ectopic 1α-hydroxylase, therefore, leads to hypercalcaemia due to increased calcitriol generation.

# Part 2

# Physiology

# Cardiorespiratory System

## Questions

1. A 55-year-old man has presented to A&E with new-onset chest pain. He has a background of type II diabetes mellitus and hypertension. An ECG is conducted.

   Which of the following features may be suggestive of a myocardial infarction?

   A  Enlarged QRS complex
   B  Absent P waves
   C  Left bundle branch block
   D  Prolonged QT interval
   E  Prolonged PR interval

2. Which of the following is used to describe the factors affecting blood flow rate?

   A  Boyle's law
   B  Darcy's law
   C  Law of Laplace
   D  Frank–Starling law
   E  Poiseuille's law

3. Which of the following gives rise to the S2 heart sound?

   **A** Contraction of the atria
   **B** Contraction of the ventricles
   **C** Closure of the aortic and pulmonary valves
   **D** Closure of the mitral and tricuspid valves
   **E** Filling of the ventricles

4. A 56-year-old man is recovering in the coronary care unit after developing chest pain and being diagnosed with an ST-elevation myocardial infarction. He has been started on aspirin.
   Which of the following hormones is targeted by aspirin and is responsible for its therapeutic effect?

   **A** Prostacyclin
   **B** Thromboxane A2
   **C** Endothelin
   **D** Brain natriuretic peptide
   **E** Nitric oxide

5. A 40-year-old man has a pulse pressure of 42 mm Hg and a diastolic blood pressure of 75 mm Hg.
   What is his mean arterial pressure?

   **A** 49 mm Hg
   **B** 75 mm Hg
   **C** 87 mm Hg
   **D** 89 mm Hg
   **E** 103 mm Hg

6. In which ECG lead is the QRS complex most prominent in a patient with a normal cardiac axis?

   **A** Lead I
   **B** Lead II

**C** Lead III
**D** avF
**E** avL

7. Which of the following types of capillary is found within the hypo-physeal portal system?

    **A** Continuous
    **B** Discontinuous
    **C** Fenestrated
    **D** Ciliated
    **E** Keratinised

8. Which of the following mediators is primarily involved in the positive chronotropy and inotropy that is achieved via sympathetic activation?

    **A** Adenylyl cyclase
    **B** Tyrosine kinase
    **C** JAK-2
    **D** Guanylyl cyclase
    **E** Cyclooxygenase

9. A 58-year-old woman with a background of ischaemic heart disease is noted to have an abnormality in her ECG. It shows intermittent non-conducted P waves with a fixed PR interval.
Which type of atrioventricular block is most likely?

    **A** First degree heart block
    **B** Second degree heart block, Mobitz type I
    **C** Second degree heart block, Mobitz type II
    **D** Third degree heart block
    **E** Ventricular ectopics

10. During which of the following phases of the cardiac cycle does ventricular pressure rise most rapidly?

    **A** Atrial systole
    **B** Isovolumetric contraction
    **C** Rapid ventricular ejection
    **D** Reduced ventricular ejection
    **E** Isovolumetric relaxation

11. Which of the following structures is responsible for the PR interval on an ECG?

    **A** Sinoatrial node
    **B** Atrial fibres
    **C** Atrioventricular node
    **D** Bundle of his
    **E** Purkinje fibres

12. Which of the following would result in an increase in cardiac output?

    **A** Increased total peripheral resistance
    **B** Increased vagal discharge
    **C** Increased venous return
    **D** Decreased oxygen saturation
    **E** Decreased aortic valve area

13. A 65-year-old man has been referred to vascular surgery after his abdominal aortic aneurysm screening scan revealed an aneurysm that measured 6.1 cm in diameter.
Which of the following laws of haemodynamics explains why this situation is dangerous?

    **A** Poiseuille's law
    **B** Courvoisier's law
    **C** Frank–Starling law
    **D** Law of Laplace
    **E** Monro–Kellie doctrine

14. A 66-year-old patient on the cardiology ward is recovering after having an ST-elevation myocardial infarction. He has become unresponsive, and no pulse is palpable. Chest compressions have been commenced and the defibrillation pads are applied. The defibrillator records a shockable rhythm.
    Which of the following rhythms could it be?

    A  Ventricular tachycardia
    B  Asystole
    C  Pulseless electrical activity
    D  Atrial fibrillation
    E  Ventricular ectopics

15. Which of the following relationships best explains the development of ascites in patients with chronic liver disease?

    A  Capillary hydrostatic pressure + Oncotic pressure > Interstitial hydrostatic pressure
    B  Capillary hydrostatic pressure + Oncotic pressure < Interstitial hydrostatic pressure
    C  Interstitial hydrostatic pressure + Oncotic pressure > Capillary hydrostatic pressure
    D  Interstitial hydrostatic pressure + Oncotic pressure < Capillary hydrostatic pressure
    E  Capillary hydrostatic pressure = Interstitial hydrostatic pressure

16. A 33-year-old woman has a pulse pressure of 30 mm Hg; diastolic blood pressure of 90 mm Hg; total peripheral resistance of 15 mm Hg(L/min)$^{-1}$; and a stroke volume of 70 mL.
    Calculate her heart rate to the nearest beat.

    A  60 bpm
    B  67 bpm
    C  95 bpm

    **D** 86 bpm

    **E** 107 bpm

17. Which of the following best describes the plateau phase of the cardiac action potential?

    **A** Correlates with the relative refractory phase

    **B** Calcium influx balances potassium efflux

    **C** The plateau phase in the sinoatrial node is regulated by T-type calcium channels

    **D** The Na-K pump is responsible for the maintenance of the plateau phase

    **E** The membrane potential is more negative during the plateau phase compared to the resting state

18. Which of the following arrhythmias would give rise to a 'sawtooth' appearance on an ECG?

    **A** First degree heart block

    **B** Sinus tachycardia

    **C** Supraventricular tachycardia

    **D** Atrial flutter

    **E** Atrial fibrillation

19. A 74-year-old patient with a background of ischaemic heart disease has presented to A&E with shortness of breath and bilateral ankle swelling. He has a chest X-ray which reveals pulmonary oedema and an enlarged cardiac shadow. IV isosorbide mononitrate (venodilator) is used in his initial treatment.

    Which of the following best describes the mechanism by which this medication will bring about an improvement in the patient's condition?

    **A** Reduced afterload

    **B** Reduced preload

**C** Increased ventricular filling
**D** Increased ventricular contractility
**E** Increased ventricular pressure

20. Which of the following best describes Frank–Starling law?

**A** Preload is directly proportional to afterload
**B** Preload is inversely proportional to afterload
**C** Preload is directly proportional to cardiac output
**D** Preload is inversely proportional to cardiac output
**E** Preload is directly proportional to end-diastolic volume

21. What is the ratio of cardiac output between the right and left side of the heart?

**A** 2:1
**B** 2:3
**C** 1:2
**D** 3:2
**E** 1:1

22. Which order of events is correct regarding the cardiac cycle?

**1.** Ventricles repolarise
**2.** S1 sound is heard
**3.** Aortic and pulmonary valves close
**4.** Isovolumetric relaxation of the ventricles
**5.** P wave on ECG
**6.** Isotonic contraction of the ventricles

**A** $2 \rightarrow 5 \rightarrow 3 \rightarrow 4 \rightarrow 6 \rightarrow 1$
**B** $2 \rightarrow 5 \rightarrow 6 \rightarrow 3 \rightarrow 1 \rightarrow 4$
**C** $5 \rightarrow 2 \rightarrow 6 \rightarrow 1 \rightarrow 4 \rightarrow 3$
**D** $5 \rightarrow 2 \rightarrow 6 \rightarrow 3 \rightarrow 4 \rightarrow 1$
**E** $5 \rightarrow 2 \rightarrow 6 \rightarrow 3 \rightarrow 1 \rightarrow 4$

23. Which of the following effects would you expect to see in response to a drop in blood pressure?

    A  Increased baroreceptor firing leading to increased sympathetic activity
    B  Increased baroreceptor firing leading to decreased sympathetic activity
    C  Decreased baroreceptor firing leading to increased sympathetic activity
    D  Decreased baroreceptor firing leading to decreased sympathetic activity
    E  Decreased baroreceptor firing leading to increased vagal activity

24. A 54-year-old man is reviewed in the outpatient cardiology clinic after having several episodes of palpitations associated with dizziness. An ECG is conducted, which reveals QRS complexes with a slurred upstroke. His heart rate is 70 bpm and regular.
    What is the most likely diagnosis?

    A  Atrial fibrillation
    B  Ventricular tachycardia
    C  Complete heart block
    D  Left bundle branch block
    E  Wolff–Parkinson–White syndrome

25. Which of the following best describes the sequence of events that results in hypertension due to reduced vascular compliance?

    1. Decreased arterial compliance and elastance
    2. Increased pulse pressure
    3. Arteries stiffen with age
    4. The Windkessel effect is reduced as arteries cannot stretch and recoil

    A  1, 2, 3, 4
    B  2, 3, 4, 1
    C  3, 1, 4, 2

**D** 4, 3, 2, 1
**E** 1, 3, 4, 2

26. Which of the following is true regarding the differences between cardiac muscle and skeletal muscle?

   **A** Skeletal muscles do not release calcium from the sarcoplasmic reticulum to initiate muscle contraction
   **B** Cardiac muscle can only demonstrate isometric contraction
   **C** The amount of active force produced by cardiac muscle is considerably higher than skeletal muscle
   **D** Skeletal muscles are more compliant than cardiac muscle
   **E** The relationship between force generation and intracellular calcium concentration is linear for skeletal muscle

27. Which of the following is true regarding heart failure with preserved ejection fraction?

   **A** Characterised by myocardial dilatation
   **B** Analogous to systolic heart failure
   **C** Associated with a reduced end-diastolic volume
   **D** Usually occurs following an acute cardiac event
   **E** Treatment mainly involves reducing preload

28. Which of the following is true regarding the autonomic control of the heart?

   **A** Parasympathetic fibres innervating the heart have a thoracolumbar distribution
   **B** Postganglionic vagal fibres stimulate nicotinic acetylcholine receptors in the heart
   **C** Activation of Gi linked receptors reduces cellular cAMP concentration
   **D** The sympathetic nervous input is greater than the parasympathetic input to the heart
   **E** Parasympathetic stimulation steepens the sinoatrial prepotential

29. Which of the following measures can be used as a marker of preload?

    A  End-diastolic volume
    B  End-systolic volume
    C  Cardiac output
    D  Atrial pressure
    E  Ventricular pressure

30. A 55-year-old woman is taken to A&E after collapsing at home. She has no recollection of the event. Her observations reveal a blood pressure of 88/60 mm Hg and a heart rate of 28 bpm. An ECG reveals dissociation of QRS complexes from P waves.
    What is the most likely diagnosis?

    A  First degree heart block
    B  Second degree heart block, Mobitz type I
    C  Second degree heart block, Mobitz type II
    D  Complete heart block
    E  Sinus bradycardia

31. Which of the following denotes the end-diastolic pressure/volume in this pressure-volume loop?

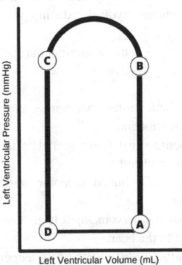

A A
B B
C C
D D
E C–D

32. A 71-year-old man presents to A&E complaining of chest pain. His ECG shows signs of ventricular hypertrophy and an ejection systolic murmur is heard upon auscultation.
What is the most likely diagnosis?

    A Aortic stenosis
    B Aortic regurgitation
    C Mitral stenosis
    D Mitral regurgitation
    E Ventricular septal defect

33. A 69-year-old man has presented to A&E with shortness of breath and a cough. A chest X-ray reveals extensive pulmonary oedema and an enlarged cardiac shadow, in keeping with acute heart failure.
Which of the following aspects of his management is most important in relieving the preload on his heart?

    A Furosemide (diuretic)
    B Bisoprolol (beta-blocker)
    C Aspirin (anti-platelet)
    D Ramipril (ACE inhibitor)
    E Digoxin (cardiac glycoside)

34. Which of the following cells is responsible for producing surfactant within the lungs?

    A Alveolar macrophage
    B Fibroblast
    C Endothelial cell

    **D** Type I pneumocyte

    **E** Type II pneumocyte

35. If a patient has a tidal volume of 0.45 L, dead space of 0.2 L and a respiratory rate of 19 breaths per minute, what is their minute ventilation?

    **A** 4.20 L/min

    **B** 4.50 L/min

    **C** 4.75 L/min

    **D** 5.00 L/min

    **E** 5.20 L/min

36. A 71-year-old man has been admitted to hospital with an infective exacerbation of COPD. He is treated with salbutamol and ipratropium nebulisers. His oxygen saturation target range is set at 88–92%.
    Which of the following best explains the choice of his oxygen saturation target?

    **A** Hyperoxygenation risks oxidative damage to alveoli

    **B** Ventilation-perfusion mismatch

    **C** Hyperoxygenation can cause respiratory alkalosis

    **D** Reliance on the hypoxic drive to breathe

    **E** Increased sensitivity to hypercapnia

37. Which of the following cells secrete antibacterial enzymes within the respiratory tract?

    **A** Mucous cell

    **B** Serous cell

    **C** Paneth cell

    **D** Kupffer cell

    **E** Goblet cell

38. Which of the following terms is used to describe a temporary cessation in breathing?

**A** Hypoventilation
**B** Hypopnoea
**C** Apnoea
**D** Dyspnoea
**E** Orthopnoea

39. A 19-year-old student jumps into an ice-cold swimming pool. The sudden exposure to the cold temperature results in an inspiratory gasp. Which respiratory centres elicit this response?

    **A** Dorsal respiratory group
    **B** Ventral respiratory group
    **C** Apneustic centre
    **D** Pneumotaxic centre
    **E** Chemoreceptor trigger zone

40. Which of the following statements best describes asthma?

    **A** Chronic airway disease characterised by irreversible bronchoconstriction
    **B** Neutrophils are found in abundance during an exacerbation of asthma
    **C** Can be caused by smoking
    **D** Treatment often involves corticosteroids
    **E** Mainly affects alveoli

41. Which of the following best describes the relationship between the chest wall and lungs at functional residual capacity?

    **A** Chest wall recoil outwards > lung recoil inwards
    **B** Chest wall recoil outwards < lung recoil inwards
    **C** Chest wall recoil inwards > lung recoil inwards
    **D** Chest wall recoil outwards < lung recoil outwards
    **E** Chest wall recoil outwards = lung recoil inwards

42. Which of the following structures is responsible for warming and humidifying inspired air?

A Nasal conchae
B Cilia
C Epiglottis
D Carina
E Adenoids

43. Which of the following would cause a leftward shift in the oxygen dissociation curve?

A Increased pH
B High 2,3-DPG
C Hypothermia
D Iron deficiency anaemia
E High HbF

44. Which of the following is a long-term complication of COPD?

A Heart failure
B Type II diabetes mellitus
C Chronic liver disease
D Chronic kidney disease
E Peripheral neuropathy

45. A young man is camping in Canada when a grizzly bear enters the camp. Instantly, he begins breathing more deeply.
Which of the following neuroanatomical structures is likely to have triggered this change in his respiratory pattern?

A Prefrontal cortex
B Primary visual cortex
C Hypothalamus
D Midbrain
E Medulla

46. Which of the following pressures is responsible for the movement of air during ventilation?

**A** Transpulmonary pressure
**B** Transrespiratory pressure
**C** Transthoracic pressure
**D** Intrapleural pressure
**E** Intra-alveolar pressure

47. A 61-year-old man is referred to the respiratory clinic after developing progressive shortness of breath on exertion over the last 6 months. This has been accompanied by a chronic cough that is sometimes productive of yellow sputum. He has a long history of heavy smoking, so a diagnosis of COPD is suspected.
    Which of the following agents may play a role in the management of his condition?

    **A** Beta-blockers
    **B** Aspirin
    **C** Muscarinic antagonists
    **D** Non-steroidal anti-inflammatory drugs
    **E** Aldosterone antagonists

48. The respiratory and renal systems are important in regulating acid-base balance within the body.
    Which of the following acid-base imbalances would you expect to see in patients with severe, prolonged diarrhoea?

    **A** Metabolic acidosis with compensatory hyperventilation
    **B** Metabolic acidosis with compensatory hypoventilation
    **C** Metabolic alkalosis with compensatory hyperventilation
    **D** Metabolic alkalosis with compensatory hypoventilation
    **E** Mixed metabolic and respiratory alkalosis

49. A 67-year-old patient with a background of heavy smoking has been recently diagnosed with COPD after complaining of breathlessness and reduced exercise tolerance over the past 6 months. He is investigated with spirometry.

Which of the following best describes the flow-volume loop that you would expect to see?

A Blunted inspiratory and expiratory curves
B Blunted expiratory curve
C Curve displacement to the right, with reduced vital capacity
D Curve displacement to the left with an indented expiratory curve
E Curve displacement to the left, with a shorter indented expiratory curve

50. A 61-year-old patient with a background of heavy smoking has developed worsening shortness of breath on exertion. He has been referred for spirometry to further evaluate his respiratory function.
Which of the following is true regarding the interpretation of spirometry results?

A High FVC is suggestive of restrictive lung disease
B High FVC is suggestive of obstructive lung disease
C High FEV1 is suggestive of restrictive lung disease
D Low FEV1/FVC ratio is suggestive of obstructive lung disease
E Normal FEV1/FVC ratio is around 0.6

# Answers

## 1. C (Left bundle branch block)

New-onset chest pain in a patient with vascular risk factors (e.g. smoking, obesity, hypertension, diabetes mellitus, hypercholesterolaemia) requires prompt investigation and management. An ECG should be performed in any patient presenting with chest pain. Features of myocardial infarction include ST elevation, ST depression and new-onset left bundle branch block.

T wave inversion may be a normal variant seen in a healthy individual, however, new T wave inversion, in a patient who did not previously have T wave inversion, is suggestive of myocardial ischaemia. Enlarged QRS complexes may be seen in patients with ventricular hypertrophy (e.g. secondary to hypertension or aortic stenosis). An irregularly irregular tachycardia with absent P waves is the hallmark of atrial fibrillation. Prolonged QT interval may be hereditary (e.g. Romano-Ward syndrome) or it may develop secondary to electrolyte imbalances (e.g. hypokalaemia). It is important to treat, if possible, because it increases the risk of developing fatal ventricular arrhythmias. A fixed, prolonged PR interval is the definition of first-degree heart block.

## 2. B (Darcy's law)

Darcy's law states that blood flow rate is directly proportional to the pressure gradient and inversely proportional to resistance. It can be denoted by the following equation.

$$\text{Flow Rate} = \text{Pressure Gradient} \div \text{Resistance}$$

Boyle's law states that the pressure exerted by an ideal gas is inversely proportional to the volume it occupies, provided that temperature and amount of gas remain constant. The law of Laplace states that the tension within the wall of a tube is directly proportional to the pressure exerted from within, and the radius of the vessel. This explains why aneurysms tend to continue to enlarge because the tension across the wall will increase as the radius increases, even if the pressure remains constant. Frank–Starling law states that stroke volume is directly proportional to preload (end-diastolic volume).

Poiseuille's law states that there are three main factors that determine resistance to blood flow: vessel radius, vessel length and viscosity. Of these, changes in vessel radius bring about the greatest change in resistance. Furthermore, generally speaking, vessel length and blood viscosity remains the same in the body, therefore, vessel radius is the only functionally relevant determinant of vascular resistance.

### 3. C (Closure of the aortic and pulmonary valves)

The normal heart sounds are described as S1 and S2. S1 is caused by closure of the mitral and tricuspid valves, at which point ventricular contraction begins (systole). At the end of systole, the aortic and pulmonary valves will close giving rise to the S2 heart sound. Added heart sounds, S3 and S4, may be heard in heart failure. S3 is caused by rapid ventricular filling, whereas S4 is caused by the contraction of atria against stiffened ventricles.

### 4. B (Thromboxane A2)

Aspirin is an antiplatelet that is commonly used in the treatment of ischaemic heart disease and cerebrovascular disease. It is an irreversible COX-1 inhibitor, which results in reduced production of thromboxane A2 by platelets. Thromboxane A2 is known to have prothrombotic and vasoconstricting effects. Prostacyclin is a vasodilator that has antiplatelet effects and is a downstream product of the arachidonic acid pathway mediated by COX. Prostacyclin, however, is primarily produced by endothelial cells whereas thromboxane A2 is primarily produced by platelets. Low-dose aspirin, used in ischaemic heart disease, will initially inhibit COX-1 in both endothelial cells and platelets, however, the endothelial cells are able to upregulate COX-1 expression to ensure that prostacyclin continues to be produced. Platelets, on the other hand, are enucleated and are unable to upregulate the expression of COX-1 to overcome the effect of aspirin.

Endothelins are vasoconstrictors that are produced by endothelial cells. Endothelin inhibitors are typically used in the treatment of pulmonary hypertension. Brain natriuretic peptide is a hormone produced in response to ventricular stretch. It increases urinary excretion of sodium and, hence, water. It has a modest physiological role; however, it is used in the diagnosis of heart failure. Nitric oxide is a potent vasodilator. Isosorbide mononitrate and glyceryl trinitrate are used in the treatment of angina as it increases nitric oxide production.

### 5. D (89 mm Hg)

Mean arterial pressure can be defined by the following equation:

$$MAP = SBP - \tfrac{2}{3} \, PP$$

As SBP = DBP + PP, the following equation can be formed.

$$MAP = (DBP + PP) - \tfrac{2}{3} \, PP$$
$$MAP = (75 + 42) - \tfrac{2}{3} \, (42)$$
$$MAP = 117 - 28$$
$$MAP = 89 \text{ mm Hg}$$

### 6. B (Lead II)

An ECG lead shows a positive deflection when the wave of electrical activity within the heart is moving in the direction of the lead and a negative deflection when it is moving away from the lead. The cardiac axis is defined as the overall direction of the electrical activity of the heart and it usually has a range of -30 to 90 degrees. In patients with a normal cardiac axis, the QRS complex is likely to be most prominent in lead II. This is why lead II tends to be used as the rhythm strip. Axis deviation can be determined by looking at leads I and II. If either of these leads has a QRS complex that is negative (deflecting downwards), there is axis deviation. Then, the direction of the QRS complex in aVL can determine the direction (i.e. upwards deflection is left axis deviation, downward deflection is right axis deviation).

## 7.  C (Fenestrated)

There are three main types of capillary: continuous, discontinuous and fenestrated. Fenestrated capillaries have several small holes within the endothelial cells that allow the passage of small molecules. The hypophyseal portal system is a site at which various hormones from the hypothalamus exert an effect on pituitary hormone secretion. The fenestrations in the capillaries of the hypophyseal system enables it to carry out this function.

Continuous capillaries are the most common type of capillary. The lining of endothelial cells is uninterrupted, thereby preventing the penetration of larger molecules. The blood-brain barrier is an example of a continuous capillary system. Discontinuous capillaries have larger gaps between the endothelial cells, thereby allowing the passage of large substances like proteins and cells. The splenic sinusoids consist of a discontinuous capillary system. Ciliated epithelium is found within the small airways and are characterised by the presence of cilia which help mucus flow. Keratinising epithelium is a type of squamous epithelium which produces large amounts of keratin. The skin is an example of keratinising epithelium.

## 8.  A (Adenylyl cyclase)

The sympathetic effect on the heart is mainly mediated by $\beta_1$ adrenergic receptors. The binding of adrenaline or noradrenaline to $\beta_1$ receptors results in the release of linked Gs (stimulatory) proteins. These Gs proteins activate adenylyl cyclase which subsequently increases intracellular concentrations of cAMP. cAMP has a number of downstream effects including the activation of protein kinase A and increasing intracellular calcium concentration. The end result is an increase in myocardial contractility and heart rate.

Tyrosine kinase is an important cell signalling enzyme that plays a role in cell proliferation. Tyrosine kinases are targeted in the treatment of some cancers, such as leukaemia. JAK-2 is a form of tyrosine kinase that is involved in cell proliferation. The detection of a JAK-2 mutation is used in the diagnosis of polycythaemia vera. Guanylyl cyclase is an enzyme that produces cGMP. Much like cAMP, it is an intracellular second messenger that internalises hormone signals. Cyclooxygenase is the principal enzyme in the arachidonic acid pathway. It is involved in the production of various prostaglandins, most notably thromboxane A2 and prostacyclin. Aspirin is a cyclooxygenase inhibitor that is used widely in the treatment of ischaemic heart disease.

### 9.  C (Second degree heart block, Mobitz type II)

A Mobitz type II atrioventricular block is caused by failure of conduction of an electrical impulse from the atrioventricular node down the His-Purkinje system. This appears on an ECG as the absence of a QRS complex after a P wave. It can be described as a ratio depending on the number of P waves that conduct through to the ventricles relative to the number of P waves that do not (e.g. 2:1 heart block).

First-degree heart block is characterised by the presence of a fixed, prolonged PR interval. This may be due to the presence of non-conductive scar tissue within the AV node. Mobitz type I heart block is characterised by the presence of a progressively increasing PR interval, followed by a missed beat due to failure of conduction to the ventricles. Third-degree heart block, also known as complete heart block, is caused by complete dissociation of atrial depolarisation and ventricular depolarisation. The patient will be bradycardic with no relationship between P waves and QRS complexes. Ventricular conduction is mediated by an accessory pacemaker within the ventricles. This operates at a considerably slower rate than the sinoatrial node, thereby resulting in bradycardia. Ventricular ectopics appear as broad, high voltage QRS complexes. It is caused by the initiation of an electrical impulse from a site other than the sinoatrial node. They are usually asymptomatic.

## 10. B (Isovolumetric contraction)

Isovolumetric contraction refers to the initial phase of ventricular contraction during which the ventricles contract against closed aortic and pulmonary valves. It is referred to as 'isovolumetric' because the volume within the ventricles remains the same and, hence, the contraction of the ventricles leads to a rapid increase in ventricular pressure. This will eventually exceed the pressure within the outflow arteries and result in the opening of the aortic and pulmonary valves and blood will flow out of the ventricles (rapid ventricular ejection).

## 11. C (Atrioventricular node)

In a regular cardiac cycle, pacemaker cells within the sinoatrial node trigger an action potential which passes across the atria causing atrial depolarisation. This is denoted by the P wave. The action potential will then move to the atrioventricular node, where it is sequestered for 0.12–0.20 seconds. This gives rise to the PR interval. This allows enough time for the ventricles to fill with blood before the action potential passes along the bundle of His and Purkinje fibres, thereby causing ventricular depolarisation (QRS complex) and contraction.

## 12. C (Increased venous return)

Cardiac output is the amount of blood pumped out of the heart per minute. It is defined by the following equation.

$$\text{Cardiac Output} = \text{Stroke Volume} \times \text{Heart Rate}$$

Therefore, an increase in either stroke volume or heart rate will result in an increase in cardiac output. As described by Frank–Starling law, an increase in venous return to the heart and, hence, an increase in end-diastolic volume will result in a more forceful contraction. This, in turn, causes an increase in stroke volume and, therefore, cardiac output.

Increased total peripheral resistance will cause an increase in afterload. This means that the heart is pumping against greater resistance and hence stroke volume will decrease. Increased vagal discharge will cause brady-cardia. Decreased oxygen saturation will compromise the contractility of the heart, thereby reducing stroke volume. Decreased aortic valve area will cause an increase in total peripheral resistance and, hence, afterload.

## 13. D (Law of Laplace)

An abdominal aortic aneurysm (AAA) is defined as an area in which the aortic diameter is increased to more than 3 cm or to more than 50% greater than the patient's normal aortic diameter. Such aneurysms are dangerous because they are at risk of further expanding and eventually rupturing which can lead to much morbidity and mortality. There is currently a screening programme in the UK that offers an ultrasound scan to check the aorta of men when they turn 65 years old. The law of Laplace is a law of fluid dynamics that states that the tension in the wall of a cylinder is directly proportional to the radius of the cylinder and the pressure on the wall caused by the flow inside. Therefore, even with the same flow, an increase in radius will lead to an increase in tension within the wall resulting in a self-perpetuating cycle of dilation, increased tension and further dilation.

Poiseuille's law relates the flow of a liquid within a vessel to the viscosity of the fluid, the pressure gradient across the tubing and the length and diameter of the tubing. Courvoisier's law states that painless jaundice in the presence of an enlarged, palpable gallbladder is unlikely to be due to gallstones (i.e. consider pancreatic or biliary malignancy). Frank–Starling law states that the stroke volume of the heart increases in response to an increase in venous return (preload) when all other factors remain constant. The Monro–Kellie doctrine states that the brain is a closed box and that the sum of the volumes of brain matter, cerebrospinal fluid and blood is constant, so any increase in one will cause a decrease in one or both of the others.

## 14. A (Ventricular tachycardia)

During cardiac arrest, the most important first step is the commencement of chest compressions and the securing of the airway. Once the defibrillator pads are attached, the rhythm should be assessed. The rhythms that could be identified in a cardiac arrest are categorised into shockable (i.e. a shock may be able to re-establish spontaneous circulation) and unshockable. The two main shockable rhythms are ventricular fibrillation (irregular broad complex deflections) and pulseless ventricular tachycardia (regular broad complex tachycardia).

Asystole is the total absence of electrical activity within the heart. It is a non-shockable rhythm. Pulseless electrical activity describes the presence of electrical activity that could be compatible with a pulse, however, no pulse is palpable. This is also a non-shockable rhythm. Atrial fibrillation is not a rhythm seen in cardiac arrest. It is characterised by an irregularly irregular narrow complex tachycardia with no P waves. Ventricular ectopics are large, broad QRS complexes that represent impulses that have been initiated from a site other than the sinoatrial node. They are usually asymptomatic.

### 15.  D (Interstitial hydrostatic pressure + Oncotic pressure < Capillary hydrostatic pressure)

There are three main forces that determine the movement of fluid between the intravascular and extravascular compartment. Capillary hydrostatic pressure will push some of the fluid from the vessels into the interstitium. Some of this fluid will return to the blood vessels due to the effect of interstitial hydrostatic pressure. Large plasma proteins, such as albumin, carry a negative charge and apply an oncotic pressure from within the blood vessels, which draws water back into the blood vessels from the interstitium. In liver disease, the hepatic output of albumin is decreased, thereby resulting in a decrease in oncotic pressure. Furthermore, the impedance of hepatic portal flow caused by a cirrhotic liver results in an increase in hydrostatic pressure within the portal system. Overall, this means that the capillary hydrostatic pressure is considerably greater than the interstitial hydrostatic pressure and the oncotic pressure, resulting in the accumulation of fluid within the interstitium.

### 16.  C (95 bpm)

There are three key equations that need to be used to answer this question.

Equation 1:

$$MAP = 1/3\ PP + DBP$$
$$MAP = \tfrac{1}{3}\ (30) + 90 = 100\ mm\ Hg$$

Equation 2:

$$MAP = CO \times TPR$$
$$100 = CO \times 15$$
$$100/15 = 6.67$$
$$CO = 6.67\ L$$

Equation 3:

$$CO = HR \times SV$$
$$6.67 = HR \times 0.07$$
$$6.67/0.07 = 95\ bpm$$

N.B. 70 mL stroke volume has been converted to 0.07 L.

## 17. B (Calcium influx balances potassium efflux)

Electrical impulses from the pacemaker cells of the sinoatrial node will spread to neighbouring cardiomyocytes via gap junctions. This causes a slight depolarisation of the cell membrane which results in the opening of fast sodium channels. The ensuing influx of sodium causes rapid depolarisation of the myocytes. Slow L-type calcium channels will then open, causing a slow influx of calcium. At the peak of depolarisation, the fast sodium channels close and voltage-gated potassium channels open. Then, potassium efflux is balanced by calcium influx resulting in the maintenance of the membrane potential — this gives rise to the plateau phase of the cardiac action potential. The calcium channels will eventually close and potassium efflux will predominate. This results in repolarisation of the membrane potential. Calcium will then be actively transported out of the cell and the Na-K pump will restore the ionic balance across the membrane.

The relative refractory period is when another cardiac action potential could be triggered, however, a greater stimulus is required. It correlates with the repolarisation phase. The plateau is part of the absolute refractory period during which an action potential cannot be triggered irrespective of stimulus intensity. The sinoatrial pacemaker potential is different from the action potential in myocytes. It does not have a plateau phase. The Na-K pump is responsible for re-establishing the resting membrane potential after an action potential. The membrane potential during the plateau phase is less negative than in its resting state.

## 18. D (Atrial flutter)

Atrial flutter is an arrhythmia characterised by repetitive atrial depolarisations resulting in rapid atrial contraction. It occurs due to the formation of a reentry circuit within the atria. This gives rise to an ECG with multiple P waves per QRS complex, classically described as a 'sawtooth' appearance.

First-degree heart block appears on an ECG as a fixed, prolonged PR interval. Sinus tachycardia refers to tachycardia (> 100 bpm) with sinus rhythm (i.e. each P wave is followed by a QRS complex). Supraventricular tachycardia usually refers to atrioventricular nodal re-entry tachycardia and atrioventricular re-entry tachycardia. They result in a regular narrow complex tachycardia with no P waves. Atrial fibrillation is an irregularly irregular narrow complex tachycardia with no P waves.

## 19. B (Reduced preload)

Acute heart failure refers to a state in which the heart is unable to pump blood sufficiently to meet the demands of the body. This can result in tissue hypoxia and the accumulation of fluid. Heart failure is most commonly seen in patients with a history of ischaemic or valvular heart disease. Failure of the left side of the heart to pump sufficiently results in the backlog of blood within the pulmonary circulation, thereby resulting in pulmonary oedema. Failure of the right side of the heart results in the backlog of blood along the inferior vena cava, thereby resulting in peripheral oedema (ankle swelling). When both sides fail, it is referred to as congestive cardiac failure. The main issue in congestive cardiac failure is that the volume of blood entering the heart exceeds its capacity to pump that blood out, hence resulting in congestion. Therefore, heart failure can be treated by reducing the preload on the heart by using venodilators such as nitrates. Preload is defined as the initial stretch of the heart muscle, due to the venous return to the heart, prior to ventricular contraction. Afterload refers to the resistance against which the heart must contract in order to pump blood out of the heart.

## 20.  C (Preload is directly proportional to cardiac output)

Frank–Starling law is a principle in cardiac mechanics stating that the stroke volume of the heart is directly proportional to end-diastolic volume. Preload is defined as the initial stretching of the cardiomyocytes due to the filling of blood, and end-diastolic volume is considered to be a marker of preload. The law is based on the understanding that the stretch of the cardiomyocytes will optimise the extent of overlap of actin and myosin fibres such that more cross-bridges can form. This will result in a stronger contraction and, hence, greater cardiac output.

## 21.  E (1:1)

Although the left side of the heart is more muscular and pumps the blood at a much higher pressure (~120 mm Hg on the left compared to ~25 mm Hg on the right), the volume of blood pumped out of the ventricles on both sides is the same.

## 22.  C (5 → 2 → 6 → 1 → 4 → 3)

The cardiac cycle begins with discharge from the sinoatrial node, which results in a wave of depolarisation spreading across the atria (denoted by the P wave on the ECG). During this phase, the atrioventricular valves will open, and blood will flow into the ventricles. The atrioventricular valves will then close (causing the S1 heart sound). The ventricles will begin to contract against a fixed volume of blood (as the valves are all closed) — this is known as isovolumetric contraction. Once the rise in ventricular pressure caused by isovolumetric contraction exceeds the pressure within the outflow arteries, the aortic and pulmonary valves will open allowing the ventricles to empty (isotonic contraction). At the end of systole, the aortic and pulmonary valves will close (causing the S2 heart sound) and the ventricles will relax against closed valves (isovolumetric relaxation).

## 23. C (Decreased baroreceptor firing leading to increased sympathetic activity)

Baroreceptors are stretch-sensitive mechanoreceptors that are found within the atria, vena cava, carotid sinuses and aortic arch. A drop in blood pressure would result in a decrease in baroreceptor firing. Baroreceptor firing usually causes inhibition of the rostral ventrolateral medulla which is the main regulator of the sympathetic nervous system. Therefore, a decrease in baroreceptor firing due to low blood pressure would result in reduced inhibition of the rostral ventrolateral medulla and, hence, an increase in sympathetic firing. The baroreceptor reflex will also decrease the parasympathetic output from the medulla. The combination of increased sympathetic activity and decreased parasympathetic activity results in an increase in heart rate and contractility, thereby increasing blood pressure.

## 24. E (Wolff–Parkinson–White syndrome)

Wolff–Parkinson–White syndrome refers to a condition in which patients have an accessory pathway that can conduct electrical impulses. The accessory pathway, known as the bundle of Kent, provides a link between the atria and the ventricles. This means that impulses can pass into the ventricles via the bundle of Kent, thereby bypassing the atrioventricular (AV) node. Unlike the AV node, the bundle of Kent lacks the specialised ability to delay conduction through to the ventricles. Therefore, the presence of this accessory pathway results in ventricular pre-excitation (i.e. the ventricles get depolarised earlier than they should). This causes a slurred upstroke on the QRS complex, known as a delta wave.

Atrial fibrillation appears as an irregularly irregular narrow complex tachycardia with absent P waves. Note that patients can have atrial fibrillation with a normal heart rate if they are being rate controlled with beta-blockers. Ventricular tachycardia appears as a regular broad complex tachycardia. Complete heart block refers to a condition in which impulses generated by the sinoatrial node do not get conducted to the ventricles. This results in bradycardia with no relationship between P waves and QRS complexes. Left bundle branch block is caused by an inability of the left bundle to conduct an impulse across the left ventricle. This means that the depolarisation of the left side of the heart is delayed as it has to wait for a wave of depolarisation to arrive from the right side of the heart. It causes a broad QRS complex with a prominent S wave in V1 and an M shaped QRS complex in V6.

### 25. C (3, 1, 4, 2)

As we age, our arteries will become stiffer (3) due to a reduction in the quality of the connective tissues within the vasculature. This results in decreased arterial compliance and elastance (1) as the tissues are less able to stretch as blood passes through the vessel. The Windkessel effect is a small rise in aortic pressure after systole caused by the stretched aorta recoiling in on itself to promote the movement of blood during diastole. The Windkessel effect is dampened (4) due to decreased arterial compliance. This results in an increase in systolic blood pressure and, hence, pulse pressure (2).

### 26. D (Skeletal muscles are more compliant than cardiac muscle)

Compliance is defined as the ability of an organ to distend in response to transmural pressure. Cardiac muscle is less compliant than skeletal muscle, thus meaning that it has more of a tendency to recoil back into its resting state.

Excitation-contraction coupling in both cardiac and skeletal muscle involves calcium release from the sarcoplasmic reticulum. Cardiac muscles demonstrate both isometric contraction (during isovolumetric contraction phase of the cardiac cycle) and isotonic contraction (during the ejection phase). The amount of active force produced by both cardiac and skeletal muscle is fairly similar. The relationship between force production and intracellular calcium concentration is log-sigmoidal for both skeletal and cardiac muscle.

## 27.  C (Associated with a reduced end-diastolic volume)

Heart failure is defined as an inability of the heart to pump blood sufficiently to meet the needs of the body. Heart failure is usually diagnosed following an echocardiogram, which can assess the structure and function of the heart. One of the main measures of an echocardiogram is ejection fraction, which is defined as the percentage of the blood within the ventricles that is pumped out during a single contraction. A normal ejection fraction is between 50 to 70%. Heart failure with preserved ejection fraction (HFpEF) is associated with an inability of the ventricles to fill sufficiently prior to contraction (i.e. diastolic failure), thereby causing a reduced end-diastolic volume. This may occur due to a number of causes including ischaemic heart disease and restrictive cardiomyopathy. Stiffening of the ventricles results in an inability to fill sufficiently prior to contraction.

Myocardial dilation is more likely to cause heart failure with reduced ejection fraction. Heart failure with reduced ejection fraction may also be referred to as systolic heart failure. HFpEF is usually preceded by chronic comorbidities such as hypertension, whereas heart failure with reduced ejection fraction is usually preceded by acute or chronic loss of cardiomyocytes (e.g. following a myocardial infarction). Reducing preload is the main approach to the treatment of heart failure with reduced ejection fraction.

## 28.  C (Activation of Gi linked receptors reduces cellular cAMP concentration)

The heart is unique as a muscle as it is able to trigger its own contraction via the sinoatrial node, however, sympathetic and parasympathetic input can alter heart rate and contractility. The parasympathetic nervous system will stimulate muscarinic (M2) receptors which are Gi-protein coupled. It results in inhibition of adenylyl cyclase and, hence, a reduction in cAMP. This, in turn, results in reduced myocardial contractility and heart rate.

Parasympathetic fibres have a craniocaudal distribution. Preganglionic vagal fibres synapse with postganglionic fibres at cholinergic synapses. Acetylcholine released by preganglionic fibres stimulate nicotinic acetylcholine receptors on postganglionic fibres. The postganglionic fibres then stimulate M2 receptors in the heart. The parasympathetic nervous system predominates in the control of heart function. Experiments in which both the sympathetic and parasympathetic inputs are severed have resulted in an increase in heart rate (thereby suggesting that the parasympathetic is dominant under normal circumstances). The parasympathetic nervous system achieves a reduction in heart rate by flattening the sinoatrial prepotential.

### 29. A (End-diastolic volume)

Preload refers to the stretch of the heart muscle before a contraction — in other words, the extent to which the ventricles stretch before ventricular contraction. The end-diastolic volume is the best measure of ventricular stretch and, hence, preload. Frank–Starling law is a principle of cardiovascular mechanics that states that stroke volume is directly proportional to end-diastolic volume when all other factors remain constant. This is because an increase in preload stretches the cardiomyocytes and results in overlapping of the thick and thin filaments that maximises the formation of actin-myosin cross bridges. The clinical relevance of Frank–Starling law becomes apparent in diastolic heart failure in which an inability of the ventricles to relax results in reduced end-diastolic volume, thereby resulting in reduced stroke volume and cardiac output.

### 30. D (Complete heart block)

Complete heart block is a condition in which electrical impulses initiated by the sinoatrial node do not conduct through to the ventricles. To maintain some cardiac output, an accessory pacemaker within the ventricles triggers ventricular depolarisation and, hence, contraction albeit at a much slower rate than the sinoatrial pacemaker. It appears on an ECG as a broad complex bradycardia with no relationship between the P waves and QRS complexes.

First-degree heart block appears as a fixed, prolonged PR interval. Mobitz type I heart block appears as a progressively lengthening PR interval culminating in a lost beat (absent QRS complex). Mobitz type II heart block is characterised by a fixed PR interval with the failure of ventricular conduction after a certain number of beats. Sinus bradycardia refers to bradycardia (<60 bpm) with an ECG in which every P wave is followed by a QRS complex (i.e. the impulses are initiated by the sinus node).

**31. A (A)**

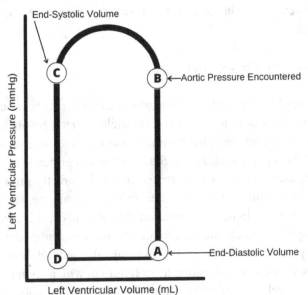

**32. A (Aortic stenosis)**

Aortic stenosis is a common valvular abnormality characterised by a narrowing of the aortic valve. It commonly occurs in elderly patients due to calcification of the aortic valve. It is often asymptomatic; however, it can cause chest pain, shortness of breath and syncope. It manifests, upon examination, with an ejection systolic murmur and a slow-rising pulse. The following method can be used to remember the different types of murmur.

To begin with, you must remember that aortic stenosis causes a systolic murmur.

Aortic + Stenosis = Systolic Murmur (Ejection)

Then if you change any one of the components of 'aortic stenosis', it becomes diastolic.

Aortic + Regurgitation = Diastolic (Early)

Mitral + Stenosis = Diastolic (Mid)

If you change both components, it remains systolic.

Mitral + Regurgitation = Systolic (Pan)

## 33. A (Furosemide (diuretic))

This patient has presented with acute heart failure. It is characterised by a sudden inability of the heart to pump blood sufficiently to meet the demands of the body. The pump failure results in an accumulation of fluid in the lungs (due to left-sided heart failure) and/or ankles (right-sided heart failure). This patient has presented with shortness of breath and the chest X-ray shows pulmonary oedema, thereby suggesting that there is a major left-sided component to his heart failure. This can be resolved acutely by giving diuretics to help remove some fluid from the lungs and reduce intravascular volume, thereby reducing venous return to the heart (preload). A reduction in preload will enable the heart to pump blood more efficiently and prevent the backlog of blood into the pulmonary or systemic circulation.

Bisoprolol is a beta-blocker that is used in the long-term management of heart failure. It is thought to have a beneficial effect on cardiac remodelling, thereby resulting in improved long-term outcomes. Aspirin is not used in the acute management of heart failure. It is used in the management of myocardial infarction. Ramipril is an ACE inhibitor that is also used in the long-term management of heart failure as it also has a beneficial effect on cardiac remodelling and improves long-term outcomes. Digoxin is a cardiac glycoside that tends to be used in older patients with heart failure. It has a negative chronotropic and positive inotropic effect.

### 34.  E (Type II pneumocyte)

There are two main types of cells that are found lining the alveoli: type I and type II pneumocytes. Type I pneumocytes are fewer in number but account for a greater proportion of the surface area of the alveolus as the cells are thin and flat. They are the main cells involved in gas exchange as they are extremely thin which allows for rapid gas exchange. Type II pneumocytes are fewer in number and are responsible for the production of surfactant. Surfactant is important within the alveoli as it prevents alveolar collapse.

Alveolar macrophages (also known as dust cells) are responsible for phagocytosing pathogenic material and debris within the airways. Fibroblasts are involved in the repair of lung tissue following damage. Excessive fibroblast proliferation can result in pulmonary fibrosis. Endothelial cells line the capillaries surrounding the alveoli.

### 35.  C (4.75 L/min)

Minute ventilation is the total volume of air that is inhaled and exhaled by the lungs per minute. It can be defined by the following equation.

$$\text{Minute Ventilation} = (\text{Tidal Volume} - \text{Dead Space}) \times \text{Respiratory Rate}$$

$$\text{Minute Ventilation} = (0.45 - 0.2) \times 19 = 4.75 \text{ L/min}$$

### 36.  B (Ventilation-perfusion mismatch)

Patients with COPD may become chronic carbon dioxide retainers over time as their body becomes less sensitive to high arterial concentrations of carbon dioxide. Many students are still taught that hyperoxygenation in carbon dioxide retainers is dangerous as they are reliant on the hypoxic drive to breath. This has since been proven wrong. It is true that over-oxygenation of patients who are chronic retainers can result in increased arterial carbon dioxide concentrations, narcosis and death. However, the mechanism is not related to their drive to breathe. Patients with COPD will have some airways that are poorly ventilated due to airway narrowing. The capillaries that supply blood to the poorly ventilated airways can detect the low oxygen tension due to poor ventilation, and constrict, thereby diverting blood towards better-ventilated airways that are better able to participate in gas exchange. If these patients begin inhaling high concentrations of oxygen, the oxygen concentration within these airways will increase despite the ventilation remaining poor. The capillaries will then detect the increase in oxygen concentration and dilate, thereby allowing blood to flow towards the poorly ventilated airways. As they remain poorly ventilated, carbon dioxide cannot be excreted via these airways, thereby resulting in an increase in arterial carbon dioxide concentration.

## 37. B (Serous cell)

Serous cells are found within the respiratory submucosal glands and produce antibacterial enzymes (e.g. lysozyme). They also secrete water and salts.

Mucous cells produce viscous glycoproteins that form mucous. Paneth cells are found within the intestinal epithelium and produce antimicrobial peptides. Kupffer cells are the resident macrophages of the liver. Goblet cells are the mucous-producing cells of the intestinal epithelium.

## 38. C (Apnoea)

Apnoea is a term used to describe a temporary cessation in breathing. A relatively common example is obstructive sleep apnoea, in which the extra weight of soft tissues in obese patients results in the collapse of the upper airways during sleep. The apnoeic episode will cause an increase in the carbon dioxide concentration of the blood. This will make the blood more acidic which is detected by chemoreceptors, resulting in the stimulation of breathing.

Hypoventilation is a reduction in respiratory rate. Hypopnoea refers to a decrease in airflow without complete cessation of breathing. Dyspnoea refers to difficulty breathing. Orthopnoea is a difficulty in breathing when lying flat. It is usually associated with heart failure.

### 39.  C (Apneustic centre)

Exposure to sudden cold temperatures will result in an inspiratory gasp that is triggered by the apneustic centre. This can result in aspiration and drowning. It is responsible for controlling the depth of inspiration during deep breathing. The dorsal respiratory group (DRG) is responsible for maintaining a constant breathing rhythm by stimulating the contraction of the diaphragm and intercostal muscles. It is predominantly responsible for prolonged inspiratory gasps.

The ventral respiratory group is involved in forced breathing. The pneumotaxic centre is a network of neurones that inhibits DRG activity, allowing relaxation after inspiration. It is considered an antagonist of the apneustic centre. The chemoreceptor trigger zone is located within the medulla and is responsible for causing nausea and vomiting in response to hormones and toxins.

### 40.  D (Treatment often involves corticosteroids)

Asthma is a chronic airway condition characterised by reversible bronchoconstriction. It usually presents in children with wheezing and shortness of breath. Bronchoconstriction is usually precipitated by exposure to allergens and irritants. It is usually treated with a combination of bronchodilators (e.g. salbutamol) and inhaled corticosteroids (e.g. beclomethasone).

The airway obstruction in asthma can be reversed using bronchodilators. Eosinophils are the predominant cell type found within the airways of a patient experiencing an exacerbation of asthma. COPD can be caused by heavy smoking. Smoking can worsen symptoms in patients with asthma. Asthma mainly affects the bronchi and bronchioles. Emphysema affects the alveoli.

## 41.  E (Chest wall recoil outwards = lung recoil inwards)

Our chest wall and lungs are opposing forces that can work together to expand and contract the lungs. The lungs have a natural material tendency to recoil inwards and the chest wall has a tendency to recoil outwards. The sealed pleural cavity acts as a connection between these two opposing tendencies, thereby enabling them to act in unison. The functional residual capacity is the volume of air remaining in our lungs at the end of tidal expiration. In this state, the outward recoil of the chest wall is equal to the inwards recoil of the lungs.

## 42.  A (Nasal conchae)

The nasal conchae are protrusions of the lateral walls of the nasal cavity. They play an important role in the warming and humidification of inspired air before it passes into the airways.

Cilia line the respiratory tract and beat in a metachronal rhythm which helps shift mucus (containing trapped debris and pathogens) up the airways. The epiglottis is a flap of tissue that prevents aspiration of food and fluid during swallowing by covering the trachea. The carina is a cartilaginous ridge that marks the point at which the trachea becomes the right and left main bronchi. Adenoids are lymph glands that are found at the superior edge of the nasopharynx.

## 43.  C (Hypothermia)

The oxygen dissociation curve outlines the relationship between haemoglobin oxygen saturation and the partial pressure of oxygen within the tissues. It has a sigmoidal shape. The affinity of haemoglobin for oxygen can change dependent on a number of factors. A rightwards shift in the oxygen dissociation curve means that the haemoglobin has a lower affinity for oxygen and is, hence, more likely to unload oxygen. It can be caused by conditions of high $pCO_2$, high 2,3-DPG, high temperature and low pH. A leftward shift would be caused by the opposite changes in the aforementioned factors. HbF, foetal haemoglobin, predominates *in utero* and it may be present in relatively high concentrations in some haemoglobinopathies such as sickle cell disease. It has a high affinity for oxygen and, hence, would shift the oxygen dissociation curve to the left. In iron deficiency anaemia there is a reduction in haemoglobin and, hence, the oxygen-carrying capacity of the blood. This can be demonstrated as a downwards shift in the oxygen dissociation curve.

### 44. A (Heart failure)

COPD is a chronic lung disease that results from irreversible destruction of the alveoli (emphysema) and chronic bronchitis. The lungs are equipped with an ability to divert its blood supply away from areas of the lung that are not oxygenating the blood very well. For example, in the case of a mucus plug, the blood vessels running towards the affected part of the lung will vasoconstrict in response to hypoxia, thereby diverting the blood towards other, healthy areas of the lung parenchyma that can better oxygenate the blood. In widespread lung diseases, such as COPD and interstitial lung disease, widespread pulmonary arteriolar vasoconstriction results in pulmonary hypertension. This can place an increased strain on the right heart, resulting in right ventricular hypertrophy and right-sided heart failure (also known as cor pulmonale).

### 45. C (Hypothalamus)

Involuntary breathing is usually regulated by the ventral and dorsal respiratory groups in the medulla. In the face of danger or emotional stress, input from the hypothalamus can override other respiratory signals and promote an increase in respiratory rate as part of the fight or flight response.

The prefrontal cortex is responsible for planned motor movements. The primary visual cortex, found in the occipital lobe, is responsible for processing visual information coming in via the visual pathway.

The midbrain is the superior-most part of the brainstem and is responsible for regulating motor movement and processing auditory and visual signals. The medulla is the inferior-most part of the brainstem and it is important in the control of vital autonomic functions — notably, control of the heart and lungs.

## 46. B (Transrespiratory pressure)

The movement of air requires the creation of a pressure gradient down which air can flow. There are a number of different pressures that are defined in respiratory mechanics, however, the overall pressure that is responsible for the movement of air during ventilation is transrespiratory pressure. It is defined as the pressure difference between the atmosphere and the alveoli.

Transpulmonary pressure is the difference between the alveolar pressure and the intrapleural pressure. Transthoracic pressure is the difference between the intrapleural pressure and the atmospheric pressure. Intrapleural pressure is the pressure within the pleural cavity. Intra-alveolar pressure is the pressure within the alveoli.

## 47. C (Muscarinic antagonist)

Short- and long-acting muscarinic antagonists are used in the treatment of both COPD and asthma. Catecholamines (adrenaline and noradrenaline) are the principal mediators of the sympathetic response, whereas acetylcholine, acting via muscarinic acetylcholine receptors on target organs, is the principal mediator of the parasympathetic response. During a fight or flight response, you would want to maximise ventilation and hence dilate your airways. This is why the stimulation of $\beta_2$ adrenergic receptors (e.g. using salbutamol) would result in bronchodilation. The parasympathetic system is active in a rest and digest stage during which the dilation of airways is not a priority. Therefore, stimulation of muscarinic receptors on airway smooth muscle results in bronchoconstriction. This is why muscarinic antagonists (e.g. tiotropium bromide) are used in the treatment of asthma and COPD.

Beta-blockers should be used with caution in patients with asthma and COPD as they can precipitate bronchoconstriction. Aspirin is an irreversible COX-1 inhibitor that can trigger bronchoconstriction by shunting precursors of the arachidonic acid pathway towards the production of proinflammatory leukotrienes. NSAIDs may also precipitate bronchoconstriction due to COX-1 inhibition. Aldosterone antagonists (e.g. spironolactone) are potassium-sparing diuretics that are used in the treatment of heart failure and liver disease.

### 48. A (Metabolic acidosis with compensatory hyperventilation)

The lungs and the kidneys are the two main organs that are important in regulating acid-base balance. The lungs can control the expiration of carbon dioxide, which is the primary respiratory acid, and the kidneys can regulate the retention of bicarbonate, which acts as a buffer. In severe diarrhoea, patients will lose large quantities of bicarbonate, thereby resulting in metabolic acidosis. In response to this change in acid-base balance, minute ventilation will increase in an attempt to blow off more carbon dioxide, and hence reduce the acidity of the blood. The increase in minute ventilation can be achieved by increasing respiratory rate or increasing tidal volume. Compensation works both ways. Patients with COPD are less able to blow off carbon dioxide via their lungs, resulting in a state of chronic carbon dioxide retention and respiratory acidosis. The kidneys will then respond by increasing the retention of bicarbonate, thereby shifting the acid-base balance towards neutrality. It is important to note that respiratory compensation can occur quite quickly, as we are able to adjust our respiratory patterns rapidly, however, renal compensation is slower.

### 49. E (Curve displacement to the left, with a shorter indented expiratory curve)

COPD is a common respiratory condition characterised by chronic bronchitis (inflammation of the airways with excessive mucus production) and emphysema (breakdown of alveoli). The collapse of small airways in COPD results in air trapping, which results in a large residual volume. This will cause a leftward shift of the flow-volume loop. As it is an obstructive airway disease, the rate at which air can be expired is reduced, which is represented by a concave appearance of the expiratory aspect of the flow-volume loop.

### 50. D (Low FEV1/FVC ratio is suggestive of obstructive lung disease)

Spirometry is a method of assessing lung function that measures two main parameters. Forced vital capacity (FVC) is the difference between the maximum inspiratory lung volume and residual volume. In other words, it is the greatest volume of air that can be forcibly exhaled after taking the deepest breath possible. In patients with COPD, the narrow, fragile airways collapse resulting in gas trapping and an increase in residual volume. This, in turn, results in a lower FVC. The FEV1 is the maximum amount of air that can be forcibly exhaled within 1 second. A reduced FEV1 is suggestive of airway obstruction. In COPD, the reduction in FEV1 is greater than the reduction in FVC, therefore, the FEV1/FVC ratio decreases. An FEV1/FVC < 0.7 is suggestive of obstructive airway disease (e.g. COPD or asthma). Note that FEV1 and FVC are usually expressed as a percentage of 'expected' based on the age, sex and height of the patient. FVC is reduced in restrictive disease as the ability of the lungs to maximally inflate is compromised. This may be due to reduced elasticity of the lungs (e.g. interstitial lung disease). FVC is reduced in obstructive lung disease but to a lesser extent than FEV1. FEV1 is also reduced in restrictive lung disease, however, it is reduced by roughly the same extent as the FVC. Therefore, the FEV1/FVC ratio may remain normal (>0.7). A normal FEV1/FVC ratio is about 0.75.

# Nervous System and Mental Health

## Questions

1. A 73-year-old woman is referred to the neurology clinic for follow-up after having a stroke. She has since developed uncontrollable and aggressive swinging movements of her left leg and arm. There is also a noticeable resting tremor in both hands.
   Which part of the basal ganglia is most likely to be affected?

   A  Subthalamic nucleus
   B  Caudate nucleus
   C  Putamen
   D  Substantia nigra
   E  Nucleus accumbens

2. Where do the cell bodies of somatic afferent and visceral afferent fibres reside?

   A  Spinal ganglia
   B  Peripheral ganglia
   C  Spinal nuclei
   D  Peripheral nuclei
   E  Peripheral plexus

3. Where does the mandibular branch of the trigeminal nerve exit the skull?

   A  Superior orbital fissure
   B  Foramen ovale
   C  Foramen rotundum
   D  Internal acoustic meatus
   E  Jugular foramen

4. A 68-year-old man presents with a 6-month history of swallowing difficulty, change in speech and reduced mobility. On lower limb examination, he has bilateral brisk knee jerk reflexes, muscle wasting and extensor plantar responses. Cranial nerves examination reveals tongue fasciculations.
   Which of the following symptoms are specific to lower motor neurone lesions?

   A  Extensor plantar response
   B  Dysarthria
   C  Spastic limbs
   D  Fasciculations
   E  Hyperreflexia

5. A 75-year-old man has suffered a stroke at home. Following acute treatment, he has a left-sided hemiplegia, primarily affecting his arm, and dysarthria. On examination of his visual fields, he cannot see anything in the left half of his visual field.
   Damage to which structure is most likely to cause this visual field defect?

   A  Optic chiasm
   B  Left optic radiation
   C  Left optic tract
   D  Right optic tract
   E  Right visual cortex

6. A 23-year-old woman is referred to an outpatient clinic after complaining to her GP about persistent headaches that are worse when lying down. They have progressively worsened over the past 6 months. On examination, it is noted that, when asked to shift her gaze to the right, she develops double vision, and her right eye is unable to move past the midline.
What is the most likely diagnosis?

    **A** Third nerve palsy
    **B** Fourth nerve palsy
    **C** Fifth nerve palsy
    **D** Sixth nerve palsy
    **E** Seventh nerve palsy

7. Which thin transparent tissue covers the outer surface of the eye and lines the inside of the eyelids?

    **A** Sclera
    **B** Conjunctiva
    **C** Choroid
    **D** Cornea
    **E** Tear film

8. A 67-year-old man is referred to the neurology clinic after suffering from a stroke. During his recovery, he has become very clumsy and often appears unaware of his surroundings. When asked to draw a clock, he only draws hours 1 to 6. Similarly, during a cancellation test, he only cancels icons on the right-hand side.
Given the clinical presentation, which of the following brain areas is most likely to be affected?

    **A** Left frontal lobe
    **B** Right frontal lobe
    **C** Left parietal lobe
    **D** Right parietal lobe
    **E** Right occipital lobe

9. Which of these cells maintains the blood-brain barrier and releases neurotrophic factors within the CNS?

    **A** Astrocytes
    **B** Ependymal cells
    **C** Schwann cells
    **D** Oligodendrocytes
    **E** Microglial cells

10. A 56-year-old man has developed a marked change in his personality following a stroke 2 months earlier. He has a tendency to inappropriate behaviour in social situations and he has ongoing weakness in his left leg.
    Which cerebral artery is likely to have been implicated in this stroke?

    **A** Left anterior cerebral artery
    **B** Right anterior cerebral artery
    **C** Left middle cerebral artery
    **D** Right middle cerebral artery
    **E** Right posterior cerebral artery

11. A 25-year-old woman is seen in the neurology clinic after developing a sudden blurring in her vision which resolved without intervention. 3 months earlier, she had a similar episode when she developed a tingling sensation in her lower left leg which also resolved spontaneously. An MRI scan of her brain and spine revealed hyperintense areas in the periventricular white matter with lesions along her spinal cord.
    Given the most likely diagnosis, which of the following statements is true?

    **A** Peripheral motor neurones have undergone significant demyelination
    **B** There is a loss of Schwann cells in the central nervous system

**C** There is an increase in the number of astrocytes within the CNS white matter resulting in axonal loss

**D** Peripheral motor conduction time will be increased

**E** There is over-activation of microglial cells within the CNS, leading to degradation of myelin within grey matter

12. Which of the following statements best describes the sympathetic outflow to the heart?

**A** Sympathetic postganglionic fibres that innervate the heart are shorter than the parasympathetic postganglionic fibres

**B** Sympathetic preganglionic fibres enter through the gray ramus communicans into the sympathetic chain of ganglia

**C** Preganglionic fibres synapse with postganglionic cell bodies within the cardiac plexus

**D** Postganglionic efferent fibres from the ganglia travel to the heart and vasculature through the sympathetic cardiac nerves

**E** Myelinated postganglionic fibres leave the sympathetic chain of ganglia through the gray ramus communicans

13. Which connective tissue layer surrounds individual peripheral nerve fascicles?

**A** Epineurium

**B** Endoneurium

**C** Perineurium

**D** Perimysium

**E** Epimysium

14. Which part of the ventricular system closely relates to the midbrain?

**A** Fourth ventricle

**B** Third ventricle

**C** Cerebral aqueduct

   **D** Lateral ventricles
   **E** Interventricular foramen

15. A 72-year-old man has had a stroke involving the posterior cerebral artery. Which of the following parts of the brain is most likely to be affected?

   **A** Primary motor cortex
   **B** Primary auditory cortex
   **C** Primary somatosensory cortex
   **D** Primary visual cortex
   **E** Broca's area

16. What structure lies immediately superior to the pituitary gland?

   **A** Hypothalamus
   **B** Cerebellum
   **C** Optic radiation
   **D** Sella turcica
   **E** Medulla oblongata

17. A 53-year-old woman has had a stroke which has left her with impaired vision. She cannot see anything in the right half of her visual field, but her central vision is intact. She also has trouble recognising common objects.
   Which of the following lobes is most likely to be affected by her stroke?

   **A** Frontal lobe
   **B** Occipital lobe
   **C** Temporal lobe
   **D** Parietal lobe
   **E** Cerebellum

18. Which of these structures can be defined as the central grey matter of the brainstem on either side of the ventricular system?

**A** Pineal gland
**B** Tectum
**C** Optic chiasm
**D** Tegmentum
**E** Superior colliculus

19. How many of the following statements are correct about epilepsy and its treatment?

   **1.** Diazepam works independently of GABA receptors
   **2.** Epilepsy is associated with excess glutamate present with the synaptic cleft and a dysfunctional GABA inhibitory system
   **3.** Glial cells can resynthesise GABA by the action of glutamic acid decarboxylase
   **4.** Tiagabine inhibits GABA reuptake proteins, enhancing GABAergic transmission
   **5.** NMDA receptors enable slow excitatory transmission, allowing only intracellular calcium influx

   **A** 1
   **B** 2
   **C** 3
   **D** 4
   **E** 5

20. Which of the following receptors would induce the slowest response?

   **A** $\beta_2$ adrenergic
   **B** NMDA
   **C** GABA
   **D** AMPA
   **E** Nicotinic

21. Which process occurs during neurotransmitter release at a neuromuscular junction?

    **A** The influx of sodium ions through voltage-gated sodium channels stimulates vesicle exocytosis

    **B** Choline is taken up into the postsynaptic terminal by choline reuptake proteins

    **C** Acetylcholinesterase within the synaptic cleft hydrolyse acetylcholine into choline and acetyl CoA

    **D** Synaptic vesicles fuse with the presynaptic membrane by the action of intrinsic vesicular transporters

    **E** Acetylcholine binds to muscarinic receptors, resulting in postsynaptic membrane depolarisation

22. Which of these cranial nerves emerge from the open (upper) part of the medulla?

    **A** Vestibulocochlear, glossopharyngeal and vagus nerves

    **B** Vagus, hypoglossal and accessory nerves

    **C** Hypoglossal, vagus and glossopharyngeal nerves

    **D** Facial, vestibulocochlear and glossopharyngeal nerves

    **E** Glossopharyngeal, trochlear, and hypoglossal nerves

23. A 72-year-old woman visits her GP after experiencing several episodes of vertigo over the past few weeks. She has noted that it seems to be triggered by standing from a seated position. The disturbances last about 20 seconds and resolve soon after she sits back down. A cranial nerve examination reveals no abnormalities.
Which vestibular structure is most likely to be affected?

    **A** Utricle

    **B** Saccule

    **C** Anterior semi-circular canal

    **D** Posterior semi-circular canal

    **E** Lateral semi-circular canal

24. Which of the following statements describes how sound waves are transduced into electrical impulses?

A Low-frequency vibrations are tonotopically detected by frequency-sensitive cells at the apex of the basilar membrane

B Vibrations move the stereocilia and induce contraction of the inner hair cells which are in contact with the tectorial membrane

C Stereocilium deflections cause potassium ion influx and membrane depolarisation

D The organ of Corti in the scala vestibuli transduces vibrations into electrical impulses

E The cochlear nerve transmits electrical impulses contralaterally to the cochlear nuclei

25. An 83-year-old woman is referred to the memory clinic by the GP after her husband reported that she is becoming more and more confused. She often gets disorientated when she leaves the house and forgets what she has done earlier that day. During the consultation, it becomes apparent that she has difficulty naming people and objects. A diagnosis of Alzheimer's dementia is suspected.

How many of the following statements are correct about the pathophysiology of Alzheimer's dementia?

1. Tau hyperphosphorylation triggered by amyloid proteins form extracellular filamentous neuro-fibrillary tangles
2. There is aberrant cleavage of amyloid precursor protein by amyloid secretase resulting in a surplus of amyloid beta
3. Neurofibrillary tangles lead to hippocampal atrophy and the degeneration of cholinergic nuclei
4. There are aberrant deposits of alpha-synuclein proteins
5. Involves neuronal atrophy of the frontal and temporal lobes due to phosphorylated tau and transactive response TDP-43

A All of the above
B 4
C 3

**D** 2

**E** 1

26. A 32-year-old man is under the care of the community psychiatry team as he has recently been diagnosed with paranoid schizophrenia. He has been started on an antipsychotic called olanzapine, which is a dopamine antagonist.
Which of the following side-effects is associated with olanzapine?

   **A** Heavy periods
   **B** Gynaecomastia
   **C** Weight loss
   **D** Urinary incontinence
   **E** Spasticity

27. A 10-year-old boy is referred to the neurologist after developing a persistent headache that has lasted 3 months. It is worse when coughing and lying down. An MRI reveals descent of the cerebellar tonsil through the foramen magnum with intense meningeal enhancement. Which of the following is the most likely diagnosis?

   **A** Astrocytoma
   **B** Meningitis
   **C** Low-pressure headache
   **D** Idiopathic intracranial hypertension
   **E** Chiari malformation

28. Which neural pathway is responsible for the motor innervation of axial muscles of the trunk?

   **A** Corticobulbar tract
   **B** Anterior corticospinal tract
   **C** Lateral corticospinal tract
   **D** Reticulospinal tract
   **E** Tectospinal tract

29. A trauma call is put out for a 23-year-old man who has been stabbed in the groin. The stab wound has bisected his femoral artery leading to the loss of a considerable volume of blood and the development of hypovolaemic shock.

    Which of the following receptors within the adrenal medulla will be activated in response to this state?

    **A** $\alpha_1$ adrenergic receptor
    **B** $\beta_1$ adrenergic receptor
    **C** $\beta_2$ adrenergic receptor
    **D** Nicotinic receptor
    **E** Muscarinic receptor

30. A 27-year-old woman is referred to the neurology clinic by her GP after suffering from frequent headaches for the past 6 months. The headaches typically arise over her left eye and are described as throbbing in nature. They typically last around 2 hours and settle after she lies down in a dark room.

    Given the most likely diagnosis, which of the following treatments can be used to prevent recurrence of these headaches?

    **A** Dexamethasone
    **B** Metoclopramide
    **C** Ibuprofen
    **D** Sumatriptan
    **E** Amitriptyline

31. Which artery is formed by the coming together of the two vertebral arteries?

    **A** Anterior cerebral artery
    **B** Middle cerebral artery
    **C** Posterior cerebral artery
    **D** Basilar artery
    **E** Posterior inferior communicating artery

32. Which of the following glossopharyngeal nerve nuclei are responsible for taste sensation from the posterior ⅓ of the tongue?

    A  Spinal nucleus
    B  Nucleus solitarius
    C  Nucleus ambiguous
    D  Inferior salivatory nucleus
    E  Superior salivatory nucleus

33. Which of the following best describes the state of voltage-gated sodium ion channels during the relative refractory period following an action potential?

    A  Both activation and inactivation gates are closed
    B  Activation gate is open but the inactivation gate is closed
    C  Activation gate is closed but the inactivation gate is open
    D  Both the activation and inactivation gates are open
    E  No action potential can be generated irrespective of the stimulus intensity

34. How many pairs of spinal nerves arise from the cervical spine?

    A  5
    B  7
    C  8
    D  12
    E  31

35. A 38-year-old man involved in a high-speed road traffic accident is rushed to A&E. An MRI of the spinal cord reveals a right hemisection at the mid-thoracic level.
    Given the nature of the spinal cord injury, which of the following manifestations is most likely?

    A  Paralysis in the left leg, loss of pain and temperature in the right leg

**B** Paralysis in the left leg, loss of fine touch and proprioception in the right leg

**C** Loss of fine touch and pain sensation in the left leg

**D** Paralysis in the right leg, loss of pain and temperature in the left leg

**E** Paralysis in the right leg, loss of proprioception and fine touch in the left leg

36. Where do second-order spinothalamic neurones terminate?

**A** Dorsal horn of the spinal cord

**B** Medullary pyramids

**C** Thalamus

**D** Hypothalamus

**E** Cingulate gyrus

37. Which of the following factors would not cause a reduction in conduction velocity?

**A** Demyelination

**B** Increased axon diameter

**C** Increased pressure on the nerve bundles

**D** Peripheral neuropathy

**E** Hypothermia

38. Which of the following structures is responsible for the reabsorption of cerebrospinal fluid?

**A** Third ventricle

**B** Fourth ventricle

**C** Choroid plexus

**D** Superior sagittal sinus

**E** Cerebral aqueduct

39. Which of the following correctly shows the afferent and efferent limbs of the lacrimation reflex, respectively?

    **A** CN V (1), CN VII
    **B** CN V (2), CN VII
    **C** CN VII, CN V (1)
    **D** CN VII, CN V (2)
    **E** CN II, CN III

40. Which neural pathway is responsible for transmitting temperature and crude touch sensation?

    **A** Corticospinal tract
    **B** Spinothalamic tract
    **C** Dorsal column (fasciculus gracilis)
    **D** Dorsal column (fasciculus cuneatus)
    **E** Vestibulospinal tract

41. Which of the following is an effect of $\alpha_1$ adrenergic receptor stimulation?

    **A** Increased heart rate and contractility
    **B** Bronchodilation
    **C** Relaxation of the detrusor muscle
    **D** Increased insulin release
    **E** Vasoconstriction

42. Which of the following cranial nerves does not have any parasympathetic function?

    **A** CN III
    **B** CN V
    **C** CN VII
    **D** CN IX
    **E** CN X

43. An 18-year-old man visits his optician with complaints about his vision. He has noticed that he struggles to focus on objects in the distance, however, he is able to read a book without any issues.

Which of the following best describes how this refractive error should be corrected?

    **A** Correction with convex lens, converging rays to a focal point

    **B** Correction with convex lens, diverging rays outward from a virtual focal point

    **C** Correction with concave lens, diverging rays outward from a virtual focal point

    **D** Correction with concave lens, converging rays to a focal point

    **E** Lens replacement

44. A 53-year-old man is seen in the outpatient neurology clinic after concerns were raised about his behaviour. Over the preceding year, he has become progressively more dishevelled, often forgetting to shower for days at a time. He has also developed a tendency to make offensive and obscene comments which are very out of character for him.

    Which of the following is the most likely diagnosis?

    **A** Frontotemporal dementia

    **B** Alzheimer's dementia

    **C** Dementia with Lewy bodies

    **D** Vascular dementia

    **E** Mixed dementia

45. Which of the following is true regarding the transmission of visual information by the retina?

    **A** Peripheral rod photoreceptor cells within the retina detect scotopic light synapsing with second-order bipolar neurones

    **B** Photon interactions within the discs of rod photoreceptors cause the dissociation of iodopsin to trans-retinal and opsin

    **C** The fovea contains the highest concentrations of rod photoreceptor cells sensitive to photopic light

    **D** Multiple central cone photoreceptor cells within the neuroretina converge with a single bipolar neurone

    **E** Cone photoreceptor cells have varying peak wavelength intensities

46. A 54-year-old man attends an outpatient neurology appointment after becoming increasingly clumsy and developing an abnormal gait. On examination, he is unsteady when he walks and keeps his feet wide apart. Furthermore, his speech is slurred, and nystagmus is demonstrable on lateral gaze.

    Damage to which of the following brain areas is likely to result in these signs and symptoms?

    **A** Premotor cortex
    **B** Primary motor cortex
    **C** Basal ganglia
    **D** Medulla
    **E** Cerebellum

47. A 22-year-old woman presents to her GP with her friend to discuss some recent behavioural changes. Over the past 2 weeks, she has had several eruptions of laughter and increasing irritability. She has slept very little as she has been staying up at night to write her autobiography which, she believes, will be a bestseller. She has a background of depression and is being treated with sertraline.

    What is the most likely diagnosis?

    **A** Bipolar affective disorder type I
    **B** Bipolar affective disorder type II
    **C** Hypomanic episode
    **D** Unspecified bipolar disorder
    **E** Major depressive disorder

48. Which of the following is a positive symptom of schizophrenia?

    **A** Hallucinations
    **B** Apathy
    **C** Social withdrawal
    **D** Poverty of speech
    **E** Anhedonia

49. An 81-year-old woman has been brought into hospital after being found wandering on the streets. She appears dishevelled and thinks that she is in Normandy and that the year is 1944. She is noted to be smelling strongly of urine and has wet herself.
What is the most likely diagnosis?

    **A** Dissociative fugue
    **B** Schizophrenia
    **C** Delirium
    **D** Alzheimer's dementia
    **E** Dementia with Lewy bodies

50. Which of these synapses are a connection between presynaptic axon terminals and a postsynaptic neuronal dendrite?

    **A** Axoextracellular
    **B** Axoaxonic
    **C** Axodendritic
    **D** Axosecretory
    **E** Axosomatic

# Answers

## 1. A (Subthalamic nucleus)

This vignette describes a patient who has had a stroke and has developed hemiballismus (a basal ganglia syndrome characterised by aggressive involuntary limb movements). They are caused by injury to the subthalamic nucleus of the basal ganglia, usually due to a stroke. The damaged subthalamic nucleus will discharge signals down the motor tracts to the contralateral skeletal muscles resulting in uncontrollable swinging of the limbs. In normal physiology, the subthalamic nucleus regulates motor function and is connected to the internal globus pallidus.

The caudate and putamen are also involved in the regulation of voluntary movement. Huntington's disease, an inherited neurodegenerative condition associated with choreiform movements, is caused by the degeneration of neurones within the striatum (caudate and putamen). The substantia nigra is a dopaminergic nucleus located within the midbrain. Parkinson's disease is caused by loss of dopaminergic neurones within the substantia nigra. The nucleus accumbens is a part of the brain's inbuilt reward system.

## 2. A (Spinal ganglia)

Somatic afferent fibres relay sensory information to the spinal ganglia. As it is part of the peripheral nervous system, the cell bodies will reside within ganglia rather than cell bodies. Visceral afferent fibres relay sensory information, including pain reflexes from internal organs. Visceral efferent nerves synapse in a peripheral ganglion.

## 3. B (Foramen ovale)

The trigeminal nerve has three main divisions: ophthalmic (V1), mandibular (V2) and maxillary (V3). The mandibular branch of the trigeminal nerve exits the skull via the foramen ovale.

Cranial nerves III, IV, the ophthalmic branch of V and VI exit the skull via the superior orbital fissure. The maxillary branch of the trigeminal exits the skull via the foramen rotundum. Cranial nerves VII and VIII exit via the internal acoustic meatus. Cranial nerves IX, X and XI exit via the jugular foramen.

## 4.  D (Fasciculations)

The progressive onset of both upper and lower motor neurone signs is suggestive of amyotrophic lateral sclerosis, which is the most common subtype of motor neurone disease. Upper motor neurone signs are caused by damage to the upper motor neurones as they extend from the primary motor cortex via the pyramids of the medulla and down the corticospinal tract. Upper motor neurone signs include hyperreflexia, hypertonia, extensor plantar responses and pronator drift.

Lower motor neurones extend from the anterior horn of the spinal cord, where they synapse with upper motor neurones, to the neuromuscular junction. Features of lower motor neurone damage include muscle wasting, hypotonia, hyporeflexia, fasciculations and fibrillations.

## 5.  D (Right optic tract)

Loss of half of the visual field (homonymous hemianopia) is often associated with strokes involving the middle cerebral artery (MCA). The MCA supplies the part of the temporal lobe containing the optic tract, thereby resulting in a contralateral homonymous hemianopia. Furthermore, the MCA also supplies the primary motor cortex, so is likely to cause a contralateral hemiplegia.

A lesion affecting the optic chiasm would cause bitemporal hemianopia (as this is the site at which fibres from the nasal aspect of the retina will decussate). Optic radiations run from the lateral geniculate nucleus to the primary visual cortex in two branches. Fibres from the superior aspect of the retina (i.e. inferior aspect of the visual field) travel in the parietal lobe whilst fibres from the inferior aspect of the retina travel through the temporal lobe. Disruptions of one of the branches of the optic radiation will cause a quadrantanopia. The primary visual cortex is found in the occipital lobe and would not be affected by an MCA stroke. Furthermore, due to the dual blood supply of the part of the occipital lobe responsible for central vision, strokes affecting the posterior circulation of the brain will cause homonymous hemianopia with macular sparing.

## 6.  D (Sixth nerve palsy)

A persistent and progressive headache that is worse when lying down is an important presentation to investigate further as it could be suggestive of an intracranial space-occupying lesion such as a brain tumour. An inability to abduct an eye is caused by damage to the sixth cranial nerve (abducens) which innervates the lateral rectus muscle. Of all the nerves supplying extraocular muscles, the abducens has the longest intracranial course and, hence, is most susceptible to disruptions by various forms of intracranial pathology. The discordance of eye movements would result in 'double vision'.

The third nerve (oculomotor) innervates all the extraocular muscles except the superior oblique (fourth nerve) and lateral rectus (sixth nerve). Third nerve palsy results in an eye that is abducted and infraducted (i.e. 'down and out'). Fourth nerve palsy will manifest as an eye that is deviated superiorly and nasally. The fifth nerve (trigeminal) provides sensory innervation to the face and motor innervation of the muscles of mastication. A fifth nerve palsy would cause facial numbness. The seventh nerve (facial) provides motor innervation to the muscles of facial expression, sensory innervation to the anterior ⅔ of the tongue and innervation of the stapedius. A facial nerve palsy (also known as Bell's palsy) typically manifests as a facial droop, but it can also cause hyperacusis and abnormal taste.

## 7.  B (Conjunctiva)

The conjunctiva is a thin, transparent tissue that covers the outer surface of the eye (sclera), beginning at the outer edge of the cornea. It covers the visible part of the eye and lines the inside of the eyelids.

The sclera is a dense, white fibrous tissue that provides a protective outer coating for the eye. The sclera is continuous with the cornea. The choroid is a layer that resides between the retina and sclera, it is composed of blood vessels that nourish the posterior aspect of the eye. The cornea is a transparent, dome-shaped window covering the front of the eye. The cornea is responsible for ⅔ of the eye's refractive power. The tear film maintains a smooth cornea-air interface and provides an oxygen supply to the cornea.

## 8. C (Left parietal lobe)

Inattention to half of a normal visual field is referred to as hemispatial neglect. The parietal lobe plays an important role in spatial awareness and orientation, therefore, damage to this lobe can result in the inability to process information about your surroundings. This is different from hemianopia, as the patient's visual pathway and the visual information from their entire field of vision will still be conducted to the primary visual cortex.

## 9. A (Astrocytes)

Astrocytes secrete various mediators that either have barrier-promoting or barrier-disrupting effects dependent on neuronal signalling. Furthermore, they release neurotrophic factors that facilitate the growth and survival of neurones in response to CNS damage. Astrocytes proliferate and migrate to areas of injury.

Ependymal cells are epithelial cells which line fluid-filled ventricles and regulate the production and movements of cerebrospinal fluid. Schwann cells produce myelin which encapsulates a single axon of the peripheral nervous system. Oligodendrocytes are the myelinating cells of the central nervous system; they consist of multiple projections which myelinate numerous axons. Microglial cells are the resident macrophages which provide immune surveillance of the central nervous system.

## 10. B (Right anterior cerebral artery)

The anterior cerebral artery supplies the frontal lobes and the medial portion of the parietal lobes. A stroke in this territory is associated with frontal lobe dysfunction and hemiplegia that affects the legs more than the arms. The frontal lobe is important in planning, organisation and moderating impulses, so damage to this lobe typically results in impulsive and inappropriate behaviour. It is sometimes referred to as dysexecutive syndrome.

## 11. C (There is an increase in the number of astrocytes within the CNS white matter resulting in axonal loss)

This patient has shown signs of two central nervous system (CNS) lesions which have been separated in time and space, which is suggestive of multiple sclerosis. It is a neurological disorder that is caused by progressive loss of oligodendrocytes (myelinating cells of the CNS) and an increase in astrocytes with axonal loss in the white matter of the CNS.

Schwann cells are the myelin-producing cells of the peripheral nervous system which tend to be relatively unaffected in multiple sclerosis. Peripheral motor conduction time is the average time taken for an impulse to be transmitted from the spinal cord to the muscle along lower motor neurones. This tends to be unaffected in MS.

## 12. D (Postganglionic efferent fibres from the ganglia travel to the heart and vasculature through the sympathetic cardiac nerves)

Postganglionic efferent fibres from the sympathetic ganglia exit through the gray ramus communicans as sympathetic cardiac nerves. These then travel to the cardiac plexus where they exert their effects.

Sympathetic postganglionic fibres run from the paraspinal sympathetic ganglia to the target organ and are relatively long. The parasympathetic nervous system, on the other hand, has ganglia that are situated relatively near the target organ and hence their postganglionic neurones are very short. Sympathetic preganglionic fibres enter through the white ramus communicans into the sympathetic chain. The gray ramus communicans contains unmyelinated postganglionic fibres, exiting the sympathetic chain of ganglia.

## 13. C (Perineurium)

The perineurium surrounds individual fascicles (nerve bundles).

The epineurium is the external vascular layer of the peripheral nerve. The endoneurium is the external layer covering individual axons. The perimysium is a connective tissue layer that envelops skeletal muscle fibres. The epimysium is an external connective tissue layer surrounding individual skeletal muscles.

## 14. C (Cerebral aqueduct)

The cerebral aqueduct is a channel through which cerebrospinal fluid flows from the third ventricle, through the midbrain and into the fourth ventricle.

The fourth ventricle is close to the pons and medulla. The third ventricle is close to the diencephalon. The lateral ventricles are close to the cerebral hemispheres. The interventricular foramen connects the left and right lateral ventricles to the third ventricle.

## 15. D (Primary visual cortex)

The primary visual cortex is located within the occipital lobe and is supplied by the posterior cerebral artery. It is responsible for processing visual information.

The primary motor cortex is located at the posterior aspect of the frontal lobe and it is supplied by the anterior cerebral artery. The primary auditory cortex is located within the superior temporal gyrus of the temporal lobe and it is supplied by the middle cerebral artery. The primary somatosensory cortex is found at the anterior aspect of the parietal lobe and is also supplied by the middle cerebral artery. Broca's area is located within the frontal lobe.

### 16.  A (Hypothalamus)

The pituitary gland resides within a bony depression, called the sella tur-cica, within the sphenoid bone. Immediately superior to the pituitary gland is the hypothalamus from which neurones will project towards the median eminence and influence pituitary hormone secretion.

The cerebellum resides within the posterior cranial fossa and is responsi-ble for fine motor coordination. The optic radiation is a branch of the visual pathway that goes from the lateral geniculate nucleus towards the primary visual cortex. The medulla oblongata is the inferior-most part of the brainstem. It is important in a number of vital functions including cardiorespiratory control.

### 17.  B (Occipital lobe)

A homonymous hemianopia with macular sparing (intact central vision) is suggestive of a posterior cerebral artery stroke affecting the occipital lobe. The part of the occipital lobe that is responsible for central vision has a dual blood supply, so central vision may be intact in these patients. Furthermore, the occipital lobe is important in processing visual informa-tion (e.g. recognising objects), so damage to this lobe can cause visual agnosia.

The frontal lobe is responsible for higher functions, such as planning, impulse control, and voluntary movement. The temporal lobe contains the primary auditory cortex which is responsible for processing auditory information. The parietal lobe is responsible for processing somatosen-sory information (e.g. fine touch, vibration, proprioception) and plays an important role in spatial awareness. The cerebellum is responsible for fine motor movement.

### 18.  D (Tegmentum)

The tegmentum is the grey matter found within the ventral part of the midbrain. It is involved in homeostatic and reflexive pathways.

The pineal gland is a small pea-shaped gland that produces melatonin and regulates the circadian rhythm. The tectum is located in the posterior region of the brainstem. The optic chiasm is a cross-shaped structure composed of fibres coming from the nasal aspect of the retina. The superior colliculus is a structure in the midbrain that is important in connecting sensory input with motor output (e.g. seeing a tennis ball coming towards you and coordinating a movement to catch it).

## 19. B (2)

2 and 4 are correct.

Epilepsy is defined as a tendency to recurrent, unprovoked seizures. It is thought to occur due to increased glutaminergic stimulation of the post-synaptic membrane. The increased excitability of the neurones is compounded by a dysfunctional GABA-ergic system resulting in reduced inhibitory signals. Tiagabine is an anticonvulsant that works by inhibiting GABA-reuptake proteins, thereby resulting in an increased synaptic concentration of GABA. This, therefore, results in an increase in the inhibitory action of GABA neurones within the central nervous system.

Diazepam is a positive allosteric modulator of the GABA receptor. It, therefore, works in conjunction with GABA-ergic neurones to hyperpolarise the postsynaptic membrane. Glial cells do not contain glutamic acid decarboxylase. NMDA receptors allow both calcium and sodium influx. AMPA receptors only allow sodium ion influx.

## 20. A ($\beta_2$ adrenergic)

NMDA, GABA, AMPA & nicotinic receptors are examples of ion-channel-linked receptors. These respond rapidly upon binding of a ligand. $\beta_2$ adrenergic receptors are G-protein coupled receptors. The binding of the ligand results in a sequence of phosphorylation and conformational change that results in the activation of a second messenger (transcription factor) that induces a response within the nucleus. These responses are much slower than ion-channel-linked receptors.

### 21. C (Acetylcholinesterase within the synaptic cleft hydrolyse acetylcholine into choline and acetyl CoA)

The arrival of an action potential stimulates voltage-gated sodium ion channels to open, causing depolarisation of the membrane. This depolarisation activates voltage-gated calcium channels. The subsequent calcium ion influx results in vesicle fusion and exocytosis. Choline is taken up into the presynaptic membrane by choline reuptake proteins. Intrinsic vesicular transporters package acetylcholine into synaptic vesicles. Vesicular adherent proteins assist in membrane fusion. Nicotinic receptors are found within the postsynaptic membrane of neuromuscular junctions.

### 22. C (Hypoglossal, vagus and glossopharyngeal nerves)

The three sections of the brainstem and the cranial nerves that arise from these regions are listed as follows:

- **Midbrain:** Oculomotor (III), trochlear (IV)
- **Pons:** Trigeminal (V), abducens (VI), facial (VII) and vestibulocochlear (VIII)
- **Medulla** (Open Part): Glossopharyngeal (IX), vagus (X) and hypoglossal (XII)

The spinal accessory nerve, which innervates the sternocleidomastoid and trapezius, emerges from the cervical spinal cord.

### 23. D (Posterior semi-circular canal)

This patient has benign paroxysmal positional vertigo (BPPV), which is characterised by sudden, brief episodes of vertigo. The brevity of the episodes (~30 seconds) helps distinguish it from Meniere's disease, which is another vestibular disorder that typically causes more prolonged episodes. In BPPV, otoliths from the utricle become detached from the macula and get lodged within the semi-circular canals. In most cases, the otoliths settle in the posterior semi-circular canal as it is the most gravity-dependent region of the vestibular labyrinth. Furthermore, the posterior semi-circular canal has an impermeable barrier that can trap otolith particles.

### 24.  C (Stereocilium deflections cause potassium ion influx and membrane depolarisation)

The cochlea is a part of the inner ear responsible for converting sound vibrations into electrical impulses. It consists of three main compartments: scala vestibuli, scala tympani and scala media. The organ of Corti is the main apparatus which transduces the auditory signals, and it is located within the scala media. It is surrounded by endolymph which has a high potassium concentration.

The basilar membrane of the organ of Corti is arranged tonotopically, whereby frequency-sensitive cells are arranged from high to low frequency from base to apex, respectively. Vibrations of the basilar membrane trigger the movement of the outer hair cell stereocilia. This moves the tectorial membrane into contact with the inner hair cells which, subsequently, causes the opening of potassium ion channels. This results in the depolarisation of the cell membrane and the transmission of an electrical impulse via the auditory vestibular nerve to the ipsilateral cochlear nerve.

### 25.  D (2)

Alzheimer's dementia is the most common cause of dementia. It is characterised by a progressive decline in cognitive function, including frequent disorientation and an inability to recognise previously familiar people and objects. Although the pathophysiology of Alzheimer's dementia is not fully understood, it is thought to involve aberrant cleavage of amyloid precursor proteins to form extracellular deposits of amyloid beta which interfere with neuronal communication. These plaques also trigger the phosphorylation of tau proteins. Hyperphosphorylated tau then aggregate to form intracellular neuro-fibrillary tangles. These disrupt microtubular structures and result in hippocampal atrophy.

Alpha-synuclein protein deposition is a feature of dementia with Lewy bodies. TDP-43 is associated with frontotemporal dementia.

## 26.  B (Gynaecomastia)

Many antipsychotic medications act by blocking the dopamine receptor, thereby reducing dopamine hyperactivity within the mesolimbic system which is responsible for the positive symptoms of schizophrenia. Dopamine has widespread functions across the body, so the inhibition of dopamine receptors has a number of side-effects such as gynaecomastia, amenorrhoea, weight gain and urinary retention. Off-target inhibition of dopamine receptors in the substantia nigra can result in symptoms of Parkinson's disease such as a tremor, rigidity and bradykinesia.

## 27.  E (Chiari malformation)

Chiari malformation is a congenital abnormality that is characterised by descent of the cerebellar tonsils through the foramen magnum. This tonsillar displacement is exaggerated by coughing and may manifest clinically as a headache.

An astrocytoma is the most common type of brain tumour in children. It is likely to be visualised as a discrete mass on MRI. Meningitis is inflammation of the meninges usually caused by infection. It is likely to present more acutely with a fever, headache and neck stiffness. A low-pressure headache occurs due to reduced CSF volume. It usually occurs following procedures that access the CSF compartment such as lumbar punctures. Idiopathic intracranial hypertension is a condition in which patients develop increased intracranial pressure with no obvious cause. It may present with symptoms similar to brain tumours, but an MRI will reveal no abnormalities.

## 28.  B (Anterior corticospinal tract)

The anterior corticospinal tract is a pyramidal tract consisting of upper motor neurones that run from the primary motor cortex, along the spinal cord, to the site at which they synapse with lower motor neurones. Unlike the lateral corticospinal tract, the fibres do not decussate in the medulla and, instead, decussate at the spinal level that they innervate. It controls the axial muscles of the trunk.

The corticobulbar tract is responsible for voluntary motor innervation of the muscles of the head and neck. The lateral corticospinal tract arises in the primary motor cortex, decussates at the medulla and travels down the spinal cord where the fibres synapse with lower motor neurones. It is responsible for motor control of the main skeletal muscles responsible for voluntary movement. The reticulospinal tract is an extrapyramidal tract that regulates voluntary movement and mediates autonomic functions. The tectospinal tract originates at the superior colliculus of the midbrain and is responsible for coordinating head and eye movements in response to visual or auditory stimuli.

### 29. D (Nicotinic receptor)

Shock is defined as a state in which there is inadequate blood flow to the tissues. This can result from a reduction in circulating volume (hypovolaemia). The reduction in blood pressure due to hypovolaemia will trigger the activation of the sympathetic system. Sympathetic splanchnic nerves will stimulate nicotinic acetylcholine receptors on the cell surface of chromaffin cells of the adrenal medulla, thereby triggering the release of catecholamines (adrenaline and noradrenaline) into the circulation. The catecholamines will then act through $\alpha$ and $\beta$-adrenergic receptors in the heart and smooth muscle to increase heart rate and contractility and increase total peripheral resistance in an attempt to increase the blood pressure.

### 30. E (Amitriptyline)

Migraines are a common cause of recurrent headaches. They are typically described as intense, focused over one part of the head (e.g. around one eye) and throbbing in nature. Patients may also complain of photophobia and phonophobia. Some patients who suffer from migraines may experience an aura during which they experience various abnormal sensations (e.g. zig-zag lines in their field of vision) before a migraine begins. Patients may also be able to identify specific triggers for their migraines such as caffeine and chocolate. Prophylactic treatments for migraines include propranolol (beta-blocker), topiramate (anticonvulsant) and amitriptyline (tricyclic antidepressant). Sumatriptan is a 5HT receptor agonist that can be useful in the acute treatment of a migraine. It is most effective if it is taken as soon as possible after the onset of a migraine.

Dexamethasone is a corticosteroid that may be used in the treatment of cerebral oedema secondary to brain metastases. Metoclopramide is an antiemetic which may relieve nausea that is often associated with migraine attacks. Ibuprofen is a non-steroidal anti-inflammatory that may be used alongside triptans in the acute treatment of a migraine.

### 31. D (Basilar artery)

The circle of Willis is a network of arteries within the brain that is formed by the anastomosis of several major arteries. It is believed to have evolved to ensure that the damage inflicted by the blockage of one artery would be limited as the supply from other arteries feeding into the circle of Willis will enable adequate perfusion to brain areas. The anterior portion of the circle of Willis arises from the internal carotid arteries whilst the posterior portion arises from the vertebral arteries. The vertebral arteries join together to form the basilar artery.

### 32. B (Nucleus solitarius)

The nucleus solitarius is responsible for taste sensation from the posterior ⅓ of the tongue. The rest of the tongue is supplied by the facial nerve.

The glossopharyngeal aspect of the spinal nucleus is involved in general sensation (not taste) from the posterior ⅓ of the tongue. The nucleus ambiguous is responsible for the motor function of the stylopharyngeus muscle. The inferior salivatory nucleus provides parasympathetic innervation to the parotid gland. The superior salivatory nucleus is a component of the facial nerve and is involved in parasympathetic motor innervation to the lacrimal, submandibular and sublingual glands.

### 33. C (Activation gate is closed but the inactivation gate is open)

During the relative refractory period, the activation gate is closed (since the membrane is hyperpolarised), however, the inactivation gate remains open. Provided there is a sufficient stimulus that exceeds the elevated threshold, an action potential can be triggered. The closure of the inactivation gate would be seen during the absolute refractory period where an action potential cannot be generated irrespective of the magnitude of the stimulus. Both activation and inactivation gates would be open during the upstroke of an action potential.

### 34. C (8)

Although there are only 7 cervical vertebrae, there are 8 pairs of spinal nerves emerging from the cervical spine. Five pairs arise from the lumbar spine, 5 from the sacrum, 1 from the coccyx and 12 from the thoracic spine. This gives a total of 31 pairs of spinal nerves.

### 35. D (Paralysis in the right leg, loss of pain and temperature in the left leg)

Brown-Sequard syndrome is a constellation of signs and symptoms that manifest in patients who have had a hemisection of their spinal cord. It results in loss of pain and temperature sensation on the contralateral side below the level of the lesion and loss of motor function on the ipsilateral side. This occurs because the spinothalamic tract (which is responsible for pain and temperature sensation) decussates at the spinal level at which the peripheral nerves enter the spinal cord. Therefore, a disruption of the spinothalamic tract within the spinal cord will result in contralateral loss of pain and temperature sensation as the disruption has occurred above the level at which the fibres decussate. The corticospinal tract is responsible for voluntary motor function and decussates within the medullary pyramids in the brainstem. This means that disruption of the corticospinal tract within the spinal cord will result in ipsilateral loss of motor function as the lesion has occurred below the point at which the tract decussates. The dorsal columns which are responsible for fine touch and proprioception also decussate at the medulla so hemisection of the spinal cord would cause ipsilateral loss of fine touch sensation.

### 36.  C (Thalamus)

First-order neurones arise from sensory receptors in the periphery, synapsing at the tip of the dorsal horn within the substantia gelatinosa. Second-order neurones transmit sensory information from the substantia gelatinosa to the thalamus. Thereafter, third-order neurones transmit these sensory inputs from the thalamus to the ipsilateral primary somatosensory cortex.

The medullary pyramids are where the corticospinal tract decussates. The hypothalamus consists of neurosecretory cells that regulate endocrine secretion from the pituitary gland. The cingulate gyrus is part of the limbic system and is involved in learning and behaviour.

### 37.  B (Increased axon diameter)

Conduction velocity is directly proportional to the axon diameter, therefore, the larger the diameter, the faster the impulse is conducted.

Demyelination reduces the effectiveness of saltatory conduction thereby resulting in reduced conduction velocity. This is the reason why multiple sclerosis, a progressive demyelinating condition, leads to impaired neuronal conduction and function. Nerve compression reduces the axon diameter, thereby increasing resistance to ion flow and decreasing conduction velocity. Peripheral neuropathy typically occurs due to vascular occlusion of the vasa nervorum. This would reduce conduction velocity. A reduction in body temperature reduces ion movement and, hence, conduction velocity.

## 38. D (Superior sagittal sinus)

Cerebrospinal fluid (CSF) is reabsorbed by the arachnoid granulations into the superior sagittal sinus. The superior sagittal sinus then drains into the confluence of sinuses by the occipital lobe.

The lateral ventricles are connected to the third ventricles by the foramen of Monro. The fourth ventricle receives CSF from the third ventricle via the cerebral aqueduct. CSF is actively secreted by modified ependymal cells of the choroid plexus. The cerebral aqueduct allows movement of the CSF from the third ventricle to the fourth ventricle.

## 39. A (CN V (1), CN VII)

The lacrimation reflex involves the production of tears in response to irritation of the cornea. This reflex is designed to irrigate the eyes and remove irritants. The ophthalmic division of the trigeminal nerve (CN V (1)) is responsible for sensory innervation of the cornea; therefore, it will detect irritation. The facial nerve (CN VII) provides parasympathetic innervation to the lacrimal glands, thereby forming the efferent aspect of the lacrimation reflex.

The maxillary division of the trigeminal nerve (CN V (2)) is responsible for sensory innervation of the area of skin overlying the maxillary and zygomatic bones. The optic nerve (CN II) transmits visual information from the retina. The oculomotor nerve (CN III) provides motor innervation to several extraocular muscles and the levator palpebrae superficialis.

## 40. B (Spinothalamic tract)

The ascending spinothalamic tract is responsible for the transmission of pain, temperature and crude touch sensation. The first-order fibres decussate at the spinal level at which they enter the spinal cord and synapse with a second-order neurone which travels up the spinothalamic tract on the contralateral side of the spinal cord.

The corticospinal tract is a descending tract that is responsible for voluntary motor control to both axial and limb muscles. Signals from the lower limb (below T6) travel ipsilaterally along the gracile tract of the dorsal columns, transmitting the sensory modalities of fine touch, vibration and proprioception. Ascending sensory signals from the upper limb (T6 and above) travel along the cuneate tract of the dorsal columns. The vestibulospinal tract is a component of the extrapyramidal system and is responsible for adjusting muscle tone and body position in order to support posture and maintain balance.

### 41. E (Vasoconstriction)

$\alpha_1$ adrenergic receptors are found on the smooth muscle surrounding blood vessels. During the fight or flight response that is typically associated with sympathetic activation, the stimulation of $\alpha_1$ receptors by catecholamines will result in vasoconstriction of these blood vessels and the diversion of blood towards skeletal muscle and the brain.

An increase in heart rate and contractility is mediated by $\beta_1$ receptors. The stimulation of $\beta_2$ receptors within the bronchi results in bronchodilation. This is the reason why salbutamol ($\beta_2$ agonist) is used in asthma. $\beta_2$ receptors are also important in the beta cells of the pancreas, where their activation would result in increased insulin release.

### 42. B (CN V)

The trigeminal nerve (CN V) does not have any autonomic function. It provides sensory innervation to the face via its three branches (ophthalmic, maxillary and mandibular). It also provides motor innervation to the muscles of mastication.

The oculomotor nerve (CN III) carries parasympathetic nerve fibres that are responsible for pupillary constriction. The facial nerve (CN VII) innervates the sublingual gland and the submandibular salivary glands, as well as the lacrimal glands. These glandular secretions are mediated by the parasympathetic nervous system. The glossopharyngeal nerve (CN IX) innervates the parotid gland (salivary function), which is also part of the parasympathetic nervous system. The vagus nerve (CN X) carries the parasympathetic input to the heart. Discharge of the vagus nerve will result in a reduction in heart rate.

### 43. C (Correction with concave lens, diverging rays outward from a virtual focal point)

Short-sightedness (myopia) is a common condition in which patients are unable to focus on objects in the distance, however, their near vision remains intact. In myopic patients, light from distant objects will focus on to a point in front of the retina. This could either be due to excessive refraction by the lens or cornea, or due to elongation of the globe. This error can be corrected by using glasses with a concave lens that acts to diverge the light coming from distant objects, thereby mitigating the excessive refraction of the lens and focusing the light accurately onto the retina.

If a patient is long-sighted (hypermetropia), the light rays will be focused onto an imaginary point behind the retina. To correct this error, a convex lens would be used which converges the light onto the retina. Lens replacement is used to treat cataracts (a condition in which the lens becomes increasingly opaque).

### 44. A (Frontotemporal dementia)

Frontotemporal dementia is characterised by atrophy of the frontal and temporal lobes. The frontal lobe is responsible for regulating social behaviour and executive functions, therefore, frontotemporal dementia results in behavioural changes and disinhibition. It is thought to occur due to the accumulation of phosphorylated tau proteins and TDP-43.

### 45. E (Cone photoreceptor cells have varying peak wavelength intensities)

Cone photoreceptor cells are located within the retina and are found at their highest concentration in the fovea (central region of the macula).

Photon interactions within the outer segment of the photoreceptor cell results in the conversion of cis-retinal to trans-retinal, thereby leading to the dissociation of iodopsin molecules. The ensuing hyperpolarisation of the photoreceptor evokes an action potential. This is then transmitted via a synapse with a single bipolar neurone. The processing of the signal by the bipolar neurone improves contrast sensitivity. The signal is then transmitted to second-order neurones (retinal ganglion cells) which exit the eye via the optic nerve and synapse with a third-order neurone in the lateral geniculate nucleus. These neurones will then travel via the optic radiations to the primary visual cortex.

To enable us to discriminate between colours, there are three cone cells (S-cones, M-cones, and L-cones) with peak wavelength intensities corresponding to the detection of blue, green and red light respectively. Rod photoreceptor cells contrastingly are used for scotopic vision and spatial recognition and are predominantly found within the peripheries of the retina. These cells converge with multiple second-order bipolar neurones — this summation allows for the detection of low light intensities.

### 46.  E (Cerebellum)

The cerebellum is a structure found posterior to the brainstem and is important in fine-tuning motor function. This includes regulating posture, balance and speech. Cerebellar dysfunction typically manifests with the following signs that can be remembered using the mnemonic **DANISH**:

**D**ysdiadochokinesia: inability to perform repeated, alternating movements.

**A**taxia: broad-based gait

**N**ystagmus: rapid involuntary movements of the eyes

**I**ntention Tremor: tremor, usually of the hands, that gets worsened during purposeful movements

Staccato Speech: interrupted and non-fluent speech

Hypotonia: reduced muscle tone

The premotor cortex is important in planning movements (e.g. during a choreographed dance routine). The primary motor cortex is responsible for voluntary control and is the site from which upper motor neurones originate. The basal ganglia, like the cerebellum, is important in regulating motor function. Basal ganglia dysfunction can result in motor disorders such as Parkinson's disease. The medulla is the inferior-most part of the brainstem. It is the site at which upper motor fibres decussate as they pass through the medullary pyramids.

### 47. A (Bipolar affective disorder type I)

This patient has presented with features suggestive of a manic episode. The DSM-5 criteria define a manic episode as elevated or irritable mood for at least one week with 3 or more of the following features.

1. Inflated self-esteem or grandiosity
2. Decreased need for sleep
3. Increased talkativeness
4. Racing thoughts
5. Distracted easily
6. Increase in goal-directed activity or psychomotor agitation
7. Engaging in activities that have the potential for negative consequence e.g. sexual promiscuity, gambling

A hypomanic episode is a less intense episode in which mood is elevated however it does not cause significant functional impairment or psychotic symptoms. Bipolar affective disorder type I is characterised by the presence of manic episodes interspersed by depressive episodes. Bipolar affective disorder type II is characterised by hypomanic episodes.

### 48. A (Hallucinations)

Schizophrenia is a psychotic disorder characterised by disordered thinking. The symptoms of schizophrenia can be divided into positive and negative symptoms. Positive symptoms are thought to arise due to excess dopamine action in the mesolimbic tracts, resulting in delusions, hallucinations and thought disorders.

Negative symptoms occur due to reduced dopaminergic activity in the mesocortical tracts. This manifests as anhedonia, apathy, reduced speech and social withdrawal.

### 49. C (Delirium)

Delirium is an acute confusional state resulting from an organic cause. It is common in the elderly population and causes include infection (e.g. UTI), constipation, dehydration and pain. Delirium typically resolves once the underlying cause is identified and treated; however, it may take weeks or months for patients to return to their baseline.

A dissociative fugue is a state in which a patient purposefully travels long distances but has no memory of their journey and, sometimes, their identity. Schizophrenia is a psychotic disorder characterised by the formation of abnormal thoughts. Alzheimer's dementia is the most common cause of dementia. Dementia is defined as a chronic, irreversible decline in cognitive function. Dementia with Lewy bodies is a type of dementia that is characterised by features of Parkinsonism (e.g. resting tremor) and visual hallucinations.

### 50. C (Axodendritic)

An axodendritic synapse is an axon terminal that ends on a dendritic spine.

An axoextracellular synapse is an axon with no connecting neurone that secretes neurotransmitters into the extracellular fluid. An axoaxonic synapse is an axon terminal that secretes neurotransmitters towards an adjacent axon terminal. An axosecretory synapse is an axon terminal that secretes neurotransmitters directly into the bloodstream. An axosomatic synapse is an axon terminal that projects onto a cell body.

# Gastrointestinal and Renal Systems

## Questions

1. A 52-year-old man has been complaining of burning epigastric pain and an abnormal taste at the back of his mouth for the past 3 months. It is worse when lying down and after he eats spicy food. He begins treatment with omeprazole.
   Which cell type does omeprazole act upon?

   A  Chief cells
   B  Parietal cells
   C  Mucous neck cells
   D  Enteroendocrine G cells
   E  Enterocytes

2. A 55-year-old man with a background of alcohol excess has been admitted to A&E with severe upper abdominal pain. He describes the pain as shooting through to his back accompanied by nausea and vomiting. On examination, he is exquisitely tender in the epigastrium with some bruising noted along his flanks.
   Which of the following enzymes should be measured as part of the diagnostic work-up for this patient?

A  Phospholipase
B  Elastase
C  Catalase
D  Amylase
E  Alkaline phosphatase

3. Which of the following statements is true regarding the passage of chyme through the large bowel?

A  Within the distal colon, anti-propulsive patterns dominate to retain chyme, increasing the time for effective absorption
B  Mass movement waves are initiated midway through the transverse colon
C  Chyme stimulates fast-moving haustral contraction, primarily within the transverse and ascending colon
D  The muscularis externa consists of outer circular and inner longitudinal muscles
E  The sphincter of Oddi regulates the movement of chyme into the caecum

4. A 71-year-old woman has been diagnosed with hepatocellular carcinoma following a liver biopsy. As the disease is localised, she has been deemed suitable for resection of the right hemiliver. A CT scan revealed that the tumour is located within the posterior-most segment of the liver.
Which of the following statements is true regarding liver anatomy?

A  The liver is divided into 5 lobes
B  The liver is divided into 8 segments
C  The falciform ligament is continuous with the diaphragm
D  Blood from the kidneys drains directly into the liver
E  Once damaged, the liver cannot regenerate

5. Which enteroendocrine cell secretes glucose-dependent insulinotropic peptide?

    **A** K cells
    **B** L cells
    **C** I cells
    **D** D cells
    **E** PP cells

6. Which hormone stimulates gastric acid production during the gastric phase?

    **A** Ghrelin
    **B** Cholecystokinin
    **C** Secretin
    **D** Gastrin
    **E** Motilin

7. Which of the following best describes the main role of peristalsis within the small intestine?

    **A** Prevent the migration of colonic bacteria into the ileum
    **B** Promote mixing of food with acidic luminal content
    **C** Propel a food bolus towards the colon
    **D** Enable the secretion of digestive enzymes
    **E** Promote the absorption of nutrients

8. Brunner's glands are submucosal tubular glands that secrete alkaline fluid.
   In which region of the small bowel are Brunner's glands predominantly found?

    **A** Duodenum
    **B** Jejunum
    **C** Ileum
    **D** Pylorus
    **E** Appendix

9. Which intestinal adaptation prevents the colonisation of pathogens within the gut?

   **A** Antimicrobial peptides released regularly to maintain the sterility of the colon

   **B** Intestinal flow stimulates the production of cross-reactive antibodies that target the peptidoglycan layers of invading pathogens

   **C** Stimulation of lymphoid mucosal follicles resulting in an IgM-mediated response

   **D** Para-aortic lymph nodes are a station from which lymphocytes can survey the gut microbiome and respond to pathogens

   **E** Langerhans cells are recruited upon detection of bacterial cell walls

10. The liver is arranged into functional units which enables it to carry out its functions with maximal efficiency.
    Which of the following is true regarding the structure of a hepatic functional unit?

    **A** It has a pentagonal shape

    **B** Zone 1 is at greatest risk of hypoxic damage

    **C** A biliary canaliculus is located at the centre of the functional unit

    **D** Cholangiocytes are mainly responsible for bile production

    **E** Each functional unit contains six portal triads

11. A 31-year-old woman presents with ongoing epigastric pain despite being treated with omeprazole and *H. pylori* eradication in the community. She is found to be anaemic and undergoes an upper gastrointestinal endoscopy which reveals extensive ulceration across the lower oesophagus, stomach and proximal duodenum. A secretin stimulation test reveals a rise in the level of gastrin following administration.
    What is the most likely diagnosis?

A  Gastroenteritis
B  Gastro-oesophageal reflux disease
C  Zollinger–Ellison syndrome
D  Peptic ulcer disease
E  Atrophic gastritis

12. Gastric acid is necessary for the conversion of pepsinogen to pepsin and provides a defensive barrier against bacteria.
Which of the following mechanisms is involved in gastric acid production?

    A  Bicarbonate ions are exchanged for chloride ions at the apical membrane

    B  Hydrochloric acid forms at the basolateral membrane of parietal cells

    C  Carbonic anhydrase activity in chief cells forms carbonic acid, dissociating into bicarbonate and hydrogen ions

    D  Hydrogen-Potassium ATPase within the apical membrane actively pumps hydrogen ions into the gastric lumen

    E  Histamine released from chromaffin cells binds to H2 receptors and inhibits the release of HCl

13. The modified Glasgow-Imrie criteria is used to identify the severity of pancreatitis by taking into account several patient and biochemical factors.
Which of the following is a strong predictor of severe pancreatitis but is not included in the modified Glasgow-Imrie criteria?

    A  Urea
    B  Albumin
    C  WCC
    D  CRP
    E  AST

14. An 81-year-old woman is admitted to the elderly medicine ward with a urinary tract infection. She is treated with ciprofloxacin and is

recovering well. Three days into her hospital stay, she develops explosive watery diarrhoea and abdominal pain.
What is the most likely diagnosis?

    A  Acute flare of inflammatory bowel disease
    B  Ischaemic colitis
    C  Viral gastroenteritis
    D  *Clostridium difficile* infection
    E  Colorectal cancer

15.  Which hepatic cells are responsible for vitamin A storage?

    A  Sinusoidal endothelial cells
    B  Kupffer cells
    C  Hepatocytes
    D  Hepatic stellate cells
    E  Cholangiocytes

16.  What physiological adaptation enables the pancreas to perform endocrine functions?

    A  The acinar cells are highly vascularised
    B  Pancreatic alpha cells of the islets of Langerhans form the majority of the gland
    C  Pancreatic beta cells of the islets of Langerhans secrete glucagon in response to hypoglycemia
    D  Glucagon release is inhibited by the paracrine effects of insulin via gap and tight junctions
    E  The GLUT-2 transporter is responsible for insulin-mediated glucose entry into cells

17.  A 56-year-old man has been suffering from gastro-oesophageal reflux for a number of years. He has been treated with proton-pump inhibitors and dietary modifications, however, his symptoms have persisted. He has recently been complaining of dysphagia and has undergone an outpatient endoscopy. An area of abnormal epithelium

is identified at the distal end of his oesophagus and a biopsy is taken (report below).

Histology: Presence of gastric columnar epithelium

Which of the following terms best describes this change?

**A** Dysplasia
**B** Hyperplasia
**C** Hypertrophy
**D** Anaplasia
**E** Metaplasia

18. A 33-year-old patient, who has presented with a month-long history of bloody diarrhoea and vague abdominal pain, has undergone a colonoscopy.
    Which of the following features is only found within the rectum?

    **A** Taenia coli
    **B** Haustra
    **C** Transverse folds
    **D** Diverticuli
    **E** Appendices epiploicae

19. What role is performed by hepatocytes in the fasted state?

    **A** Alanine transfers an amino group to glutamate, forming α-ketoglutarate and pyruvate
    **B** Lactate is directly converted into glucose by lactate dehydrogenase in the Cori cycle
    **C** Fatty acids are shuttled into hepatocyte mitochondria by the carnitine shuttle to undergo beta-oxidation
    **D** Transamination reactions occur, forming glucogenic leucine
    **E** Glycogen releases glucose-6-phosphate by glycogen phosphorylase

20. A 36-year-old woman presents to her GP complaining of abdominal discomfort that has been ongoing for the last 6 months. It tends to be

worse after eating spicy food and when she lies down. A carbon-13 urea breath test was conducted which revealed a positive result. What does this result indicate?

A  Hiatus hernia
B  Bleeding ulcer
C  NSAID use
D  Presence of *C. difficile*
E  Presence of *H. pylori*

21. Pancreatic enzymes are produced in an inactive form (zymogens) to prevent autodigestion of the pancreas upon release.
    Which main pancreatic enzyme is responsible for the activation of other proteolytic and lipolytic zymogens within the duodenum?

    A  Chymotrypsin
    B  Trypsin
    C  Enterokinase
    D  Carboxypeptidase
    E  Lipase

22. A 47-year-old patient with a background of alcohol excess is undergoing investigations at the hepatology department. He has an ultrasound scan of his abdomen which reveals a nodular liver with a coarse texture suggestive of cirrhosis.
    Which of the following are recognised consequences of cirrhosis?

    1. Hyperkalaemia
    2. Hypoglycaemia
    3. Hypoalbuminemia
    4. Steatorrhea
    5. Portal hypotension
    6. Coagulopathy

    A  All of the above
    B  1, 2, 3, 4, 6

**C** 1, 2, 3, 5, 6
**D** 1, 2, 3, 4
**E** 2, 3, 4, 6

23. Nerves from which of the following groups directly innervate the circular muscles of the large intestine?

    **A** Sacral plexus
    **B** Meissner's plexus
    **C** Lumbar plexus
    **D** Auerbach's plexus
    **E** Submucosal plexus

24. A 62-year-old man is referred via the 2-week wait pathway to undergo an OGD to investigate a 6-month history of worsening dysphagia. He is a heavy smoker with a past medical history of ischaemic heart disease and peripheral vascular disease. He has never suffered from gastro-oesophageal reflux. The OGD reveals a 4 cm ulcerating mass in the mid-oesophagus.
    Based on the information provided, which diagnosis is most likely?

    **A** Barrett's oesophagus
    **B** Oesophageal ulceration
    **C** Oesophageal web
    **D** Squamous cell carcinoma
    **E** Adenocarcinoma

25. Which part of the small or large bowel is at greatest risk of damage due to ischaemia?

    **A** Duodenum
    **B** Terminal ileum
    **C** Caecum
    **D** Transverse colon
    **E** Sigmoid colon

26. Which of the following bilirubin derivatives is responsible for giving faeces its brown colour?

    A  Urobilinogen
    B  Urobilin
    C  Stercobilin
    D  Stercobilinogen
    E  Unconjugated bilirubin

27. At which spinal levels do the sympathetic preganglionic neurones innervating the stomach arise?

    A  T10–L1
    B  T6–T9
    C  L1–L4
    D  L2–L5
    E  L1–L3

28. A 51-year-old man has been referred to the gastroenterology department after presenting to his GP with jaundice and widespread itching. He has also lost 2 kg of weight over the preceding 3 months and has noticed that his stools have been particularly pale during this time. Which of the following features of this history makes pancreatic cancer a more likely diagnosis than gallstones?

    A  Painless
    B  Widespread itching
    C  Jaundice
    D  Pale stools
    E  Weight loss

29. Which of the following is true regarding the regulation of pancreatic secretions?

    A  Cholecystokinin and secretin result in a marked increase in pancreatic enzyme production

**B** Cholecystokinin is released from duodenal K cells and stimulates pancreatic enzyme release

**C** Parasympathetic vagal stimulation during the cephalic and gastric phases prompts the secretion of pancreatic enzymes

**D** Trypsin exerts a positive feedback effect on cholecystokinin release

**E** Secretin release is stimulated by an increase in luminal pH

30. Which protein facilitates calcium transport through the cytosol of intestinal epithelial cells?

    **A** TRPV6
    **B** Transcobalamin II
    **C** Hepcidin
    **D** Calbindin-D
    **E** Caeruloplasmin

31. A 34-year-old patient is undergoing pre-operative assessment ahead of a liver transplant. She has decompensated liver disease following a paracetamol overdose.
    Which of the following blood test results are you most likely to see?

    **A** High albumin
    **B** High INR
    **C** High glucose
    **D** Low ammonia
    **E** Low bilirubin

32. Which of the following is an important property or function of bile?

    **A** Digestion of carbohydrates
    **B** Excretion of vitamins
    **C** Neutralising stomach acid
    **D** Excretion of triglycerides and fatty acids
    **E** Absorption of proteins

33. A 31-year-old woman visits her GP complaining of intermittent diarrhoea. She explains that it appears to be related to times when she feels particularly stressed. She would like some medication for symptomatic relief that she can use during these episodes. Loperamide is recommended.

    What is the mechanism of action of loperamide?

    A  Muscarinic agonist
    B  Beta-adrenergic antagonist
    C  Opioid receptor agonist
    D  Dopamine antagonist
    E  Histamine antagonist

34. Which protein carries iron in the circulation?

    A  Ferritin
    B  Hepcidin
    C  Transferrin
    D  Haem carrier protein I
    E  Ferroportin

35. A 41-year-old woman has had a CT scan after attending A&E with severe upper abdominal pain. Her liver function tests revealed significantly raised liver enzymes and the CT scan identified an impacted gallstone within the cystic duct.

    Which obstructive jaundice disorder is characterised by impacted gallstones in the cystic duct?

    A  Primary sclerosing cholangitis
    B  Hydatid cyst
    C  Mirizzi syndrome
    D  Cholangiocarcinoma
    E  Biliary atresia

36. Which cells lie exclusively at the base of the crypts of Lieberkühn and contain large acidophilic granules?

A  Enteroendocrine cells
B  Goblet cells
C  Paneth cells
D  Stem cells
E  Langerhans cells

37. A 32-year-old woman is admitted to the gastroenterology ward with ascites. Her liver function tests have revealed markedly reduced liver synthetic function. She is also known to psychiatry services as she is being investigated for a progressive change in her personality over the preceding 2 years. Given her age, she has marked mobility issues including a resting tremor and slow movement.
An accumulation of which of the following minerals within the body can account for these symptoms?

A  Calcium
B  Copper
C  Potassium
D  Iron
E  Magnesium

38. A 52-year-old woman with multiple comorbidities has been admitted to hospital with sepsis. She has been started on IV fluids and broad-spectrum antibiotics but continues to spike. On examination, her abdomen is distended, tense and tender.
Given the information available, which of the following is the most likely diagnosis?

A  Pyelonephritis
B  Spontaneous bacterial peritonitis
C  Cholecystitis
D  Viral hepatitis
E  Gastroenteritis

39. A 65-year-old man is invited to a follow-up clinic after his colorectal cancer screening test revealed an abnormal result.

He is due to undergo a colonoscopy to check for possible bowel cancer.

In which part of the bowel is a mass suggestive of colorectal cancer most likely to be found?

    **A** Rectum
    **B** Sigmoid colon
    **C** Transverse colon
    **D** Appendix
    **E** Caecum

40. Which of the following is associated with polycystic kidney disease?

    **A** Pulmonary cyst
    **B** Intracranial bleed
    **C** Osteoporosis
    **D** Pericarditis
    **E** Diabetes mellitus

41. A 35-year-old patient has been noted to be significantly hypertensive upon two visits to his GP. Accordingly, he was started on ramipril (ACE inhibitor) to control his blood pressure. He has a routine blood test three weeks after commencing treatment which reveals a mild acute kidney injury.

In which of the following mechanisms could explain this finding?

    **A** Nephrotoxicity of ACE inhibitor
    **B** Afferent arteriolar constriction caused by ACE inhibitor
    **C** Efferent arteriolar dilation caused by ACE inhibitor
    **D** Reduced renal perfusion caused by a reduction in blood pressure
    **E** Immune-mediated damage to glomerulus

42. A 62-year-old patient with a background of heart failure has been admitted to hospital with fluid overload. He has been given two doses

of IV furosemide (loop diuretic) to help offload some of his excess fluid.

What is the mechanism of action of loop diuretics?

A Increases osmolality of filtrate
B Increases pressure gradient across glomerulus
C Inhibits the Na-K-Cl triple transporter
D Inhibits the Na-Cl cotransporter
E Inhibits aquaporin channels

43. Which of the following would have the greatest effect on sodium reabsorption in principal cells?

A Antidiuretic hormone
B Aldosterone
C FGF23
D Angiotensin II
E Adrenaline

44. A 58-year-old man who has been admitted to hospital with COVID-19 pneumonitis has developed an acute kidney injury. His serum creatinine is found to be 216 $\mu$mol/L (baseline ~ 90).

Which feature of creatinine makes it a useful marker of renal function?

A It is freely filtered
B It is extensively reabsorbed into the circulation
C It is extensively secreted into the urine
D Production of creatinine is dependent on renal function
E Production of creatinine is unaffected by other factors (e.g. age)

45. Which part of the nephron is most important in concentrating the urine?

A Bowman's capsule
B Proximal convoluted tubule

    **C** Loop of Henle
    **D** Distal convoluted tubule
    **E** Collecting duct

46. A 42-year-old man presents to A&E with severe abdominal pain. The pain began suddenly earlier in the day and radiated from his flank towards his groin. A urine dipstick reveals haematuria.
What is the most likely diagnosis?

    **A** Nephrotic syndrome
    **B** Appendicitis
    **C** Urinary tract infection
    **D** Urinary tract calculus
    **E** Prostate cancer

47. A 45-year-old man is due to undergo a ureteroscopic lithotripsy to remove a urinary tract calculus that has become lodged at the right pelvi-ureteric junction.
What is the stone most likely to be composed of?

    **A** Cholesterol
    **B** Cystine
    **C** Urate
    **D** Calcium
    **E** Magnesium ammonium phosphate

48. What proportion of cardiac output goes to the kidneys in a healthy patient?

    **A** 10%
    **B** 15%
    **C** 20%
    **D** 25%
    **E** 30%

49. A 44-year-old woman has been referred to the gastroenterology clinic after complaining of frequent episodes of diarrhoea over the past month. She explains that these episodes occur relatively suddenly and are associated with palpitations, facial flushing and breathlessness. A CT abdomen and pelvis reveals irregular masses within the liver and terminal ileum.
What is the most likely diagnosis?

    **A** Carcinoid tumour
    **B** Small bowel adenocarcinoma
    **C** Gastrointestinal sarcoidosis
    **D** Hepatocellular carcinoma
    **E** Cholangiocarcinoma

50. By definition, which of the following layers of the gastric wall must be breached in order for the resulting defect to be described as an ulcer?

    **A** Epithelium
    **B** Submucosa
    **C** Lamina propria
    **D** Muscularis mucosa
    **E** Muscularis propria

## Answers

### 1. B (Parietal cells)

Omeprazole is a proton pump inhibitor which acts on gastric parietal cells to reduce the secretion of hydrochloric acid. This reduces the acidity of the stomach and can bring symptomatic improvement in patients with gastro-oesophageal reflux disease.

Chief cells predominantly secrete pepsinogen, a precursor of pepsin. In the presence of hydrochloric acid, pepsinogen will be activated into pepsin which can then digest proteins into smaller peptide chains. Mucous neck cells are gastric glands in the upper regions of the stomach which secrete alkaline mucus. Enteroendocrine G cells residing within the pyloric antrum secrete gastrin. Gastrin stimulates histamine release from chromaffin cells and encourages hydrochloric acid secretion from parietal cells during the gastric phase of secretion. Enterocytes line the intestinal walls, and their principal function is the absorption of water, electrolytes and nutrients.

### 2. D (Amylase)

Acute pancreatitis is inflammation of the pancreas that is most commonly caused by gallstones and alcohol excess. It usually presents with severe epigastric pain associated with nausea and vomiting. Alcohol excess can stimulate the premature activation of pancreatic zymogens resulting in autodigestion of the pancreas by the very enzymes that it produces. Two pancreatic enzymes in particular, amylase and lipase, are used in the diagnosis of acute pancreatitis as they leak into the circulation and can be detected in high concentrations in the peripheral blood. Elastase is another enzyme produced by the pancreas which is responsible for protein digestion. A low concentration of elastase in the faeces is a marker of pancreatic exocrine dysfunction.

Phospholipase and catalase are not used in diagnostic investigations. Alkaline phosphatase is an enzyme that is primarily found in the bone and biliary tree. Therefore, it is useful in the investigation of bone pathology (e.g. Paget's disease) and biliary pathology (e.g. gallstones).

### 3.  B (Mass movement waves are initiated midway through the transverse colon)

Mass movement waves are initiated midway through the transverse colon, propelling chyme towards the rectum in a sustained manner that resembles peristaltic contractions. These movements increase in frequency after a meal (gastrocolic reflex).

Anti-propulsive patterns mainly occur within the proximal colon which prolongs the transit of chyme and allows more time for the reabsorption of water. Chyme stimulates slow-moving haustral contractions. This slow movement facilitates the absorption of water and electrolytes in the transverse and descending colon. The muscularis externa is a muscular layer composed of inner circular muscles and outer longitudinal muscles. The longitudinal muscles are concentrated into bands called taenia coli. The ileocaecal valve is responsible for regulating the movement of chyme into the caecum.

### 4.  B (The liver is divided into 8 segments)

The liver is located within the right upper quadrant of the abdomen and has a number of important functions including plasma protein and clotting factor synthesis, gluconeogenesis, drug and toxin metabolism, and bile production. It is divided into 4 lobes (right, left, caudate and quadrate) and 8 segments (I to VIII).

The falciform ligament is an embryological remnant of the ventral mesentery and it attaches the liver to the anterior abdominal wall. The coronary ligament is located on the superior surface of the liver and attaches the liver to the inferior surface of the diaphragm. The liver has two major blood supplies: the hepatic artery (arising from the coeliac axis) and the hepatic portal vein (delivering blood from the intestines and spleen). The bulk of the liver is made up of hepatocytes which do have a capacity to regenerate following damage. Persistent damage, however, can result in the deposition of scar tissue, known as cirrhosis.

## 5. A (K cells)

Mucosal enteroendocrine K cells release glucose-dependent insulino-tropic peptide, also known as gastric inhibitory polypeptide. It is stimulated by the presence of high concentrations of glucose within the duodenum and results in decreased gastric acid secretion and increased insulin release from the pancreas.

Enteroendocrine L cells secrete peptide YY which reduces intestinal motility, gallbladder contraction and pancreatic exocrine secretion. It also has an inhibitory effect on appetite. I cells secrete cholecystokinin in response to the presence of fatty acids and amino acids in the duodenum. It delays gastric emptying and stimulates the release of pancreatic enzymes. D cells release somatostatin which has a generalised inhibitory effect on other hormones. It will reduce gastric, intestinal and pancreatic secretion, intestinal motility and the release of gastrointestinal hormones. It is sometimes dubbed '*endocrine cyanide*' for its widespread inhibitory effects. PP cells secrete pancreatic polypeptide from the islets of Langerhans. It inhibits pancreatic enzyme and bicarbonate secretion.

## 6. D (Gastrin)

Gastrin is released by enteroendocrine G cells within the pyloric antrum of the stomach. Its release is stimulated by the presence of food in the stomach. This action is potentiated by hormonal interactions with enterochromaffin-like cells, resulting in the release of histamine.

Ghrelin acts on the hypothalamus to induce sensations of hunger. Cholecystokinin is released as part of the enteric inhibitory reflex during the intestinal phase. It delays gastric emptying and stimulates gallbladder contraction. Secretin is released from enteroendocrine S cells of the duodenum and jejunum. It stimulates pancreatic bicarbonate secretion from acinar and ductal cells. Motilin controls the muscular contractions of the upper gastrointestinal tract.

## 7. C (Propel a food bolus towards the colon)

Peristalsis is the controlled contraction of circular smooth muscle surrounding the small bowel which results in the propulsion of chyme towards the colon. These movements are coordinated by the enteric nervous system.

The ileocaecal valve prevents colonic bacteria from colonising the small bowel. The stomach is responsible for the storage of food and the mixing of the food in the acidic environment which aids its breakdown. The secretion of digestive enzymes is controlled by various hormones secreted throughout the gastrointestinal tract. Peristalsis does not directly promote the absorption of nutrients.

## 8. A (Duodenum)

Brunner's glands are located within the duodenum and open into the base of the crypts. They release alkaline secretions that are rich in bicarbonate to neutralise acidic chyme and protect the proximal small bowel from acidic contents passing into the duodenum from the stomach. The caecum and appendix are parts of the large bowel.

## 9. B (Intestinal flow stimulates the production of cross-reactive antibodies that target the peptidoglycan layers of invading pathogens)

Cross-reactive antibodies are produced against normal components of intestinal flora. This is stimulated by intestinal flow and the antibodies are directed towards the peptidoglycan cell wall of invading pathogens.

The colon is populated by numerous commensal bacteria which are important in creating a competitive environment in which pathogens cannot gain a foothold. Antimicrobial peptides are released by Paneth cells in the duodenum to help maintain the sterility of the small intestine. Mucosal lymphoid follicles produce an IgA-mediated response to stimulation. Peyer's patches are mucosa-associated lymphoid tissue that act as stations for immunological surveillance of the gastrointestinal tract. The cell wall of pathogens can trigger the recruitment of dendritic cells. Langerhans are dendritic cells that are found within the skin.

### 10. E (Each functional unit contains six portal triads)

The liver is neatly arranged into functional units which include a blood supply, biliary vessels and hepatocytes. They are hexagonal and contain a portal triad (branch of hepatic artery, branch of the portal vein and branch of the biliary tree) at each of the six vertices. At the centre of the hexagonal functional unit is a central vein into which the detoxified blood will drain. The region between the portal triad and the central vein is divided into three zones with zone 1 being nearest the portal triad and zone 3 being nearest the central vein. Zone 3 is particularly vulnerable to hypoxic damage as it is furthest from the branches of the hepatic arteries within the portal triad. The majority of bile production occurs within the hepatocytes, however, the cholangiocytes are important in secreting water and electrolytes into the bile.

### 11. C (Zollinger–Ellison syndrome)

Zollinger–Ellison syndrome is a condition in which patients present with extensive mucosal ulceration across their oesophagus, stomach and proximal small bowel due to very elevated levels of gastrin. This is caused by a benign tumour of the enteroendocrine G cells. The high concentrations of gastrin will increase acid output within the stomach which gives rise to widespread mucosal damage and ulceration. A secretin stimulation test is often used to diagnose the disease as secretin would normally inhibit gastrin production but, in Zollinger–Ellison syndrome, you see a paradoxical rise in gastrin following administration of secretin.

Gastroenteritis is acute inflammation of the gastrointestinal tract due to a virus or bacterium. It typically presents with diarrhoea and vomiting and is usually self-limiting. Gastro-oesophageal reflux disease usually presents with vague epigastric pain and, sometimes, a cough. It results from an inability of the lower oesophageal sphincter to maintain a seal between the oesophagus and stomach. The disease is limited to the oesophagus. Peptic ulcer disease refers to the appearance of ulcers in the lining of gastrointestinal mucosa. Although this patient has developed peptic ulcers, the extent of the ulceration and the diagnostic test results make Zollinger–Ellison syndrome a better answer. Atrophic gastritis is an autoimmune condition that results in atrophy of the gastric mucosa. It can lead to vitamin B12 deficiency due to an inability of the gastric parietal cells to produce intrinsic factor which is necessary for the gastrointestinal transit of vitamin B12.

## 12. D (Hydrogen-Potassium ATPase within the apical membrane actively pumps hydrogen ions into the gastric lumen)

Hydrogen-Potassium ATPase is found on the apical membrane of gastric parietal cells. It actively secretes protons into the gastric lumen.

The bicarbonate-chloride anion exchanger is embedded within the basolateral membrane. Hydrochloric acid is secreted from the apical aspect of the gastric parietal cells. Carbonic anhydrase activity occurs within parietal cells, not chief cells. Histamine released by chromaffin cells binds to H2 receptors and stimulates the release of hydrochloric acid.

## 13. D (CRP)

The modified Glasgow-Imrie criteria take into account a number of factors including age, white cell count, calcium, urea, LDH, albumin and glucose, to determine the severity of pancreatitis. A score of more than 3 within 48 hours of the onset is suggestive of severe pancreatitis. C-reactive protein, an acute phase protein that is elevated in most inflammatory and infectious conditions, has been identified as an independent marker of pancreatitis severity.

## 14. D (*Clostridium difficile* infection)

*Clostridium difficile* is a Gram-positive bacterium that is found in the colon of many healthy individuals. It can, however, overgrow within the colon and produce toxins that induce an inflammatory response within the colon. The toxins have a cytotoxic effect on enterocytes which results in excessive fluid leakage from intestinal epithelium and patchy necrosis. The sloughing of necrotic tissue results in a 'pseudomembranous' appearance. The use of antibiotics, in particular ciprofloxacin, cephalosporins and clindamycin, is associated with an increased risk of *C. difficile* colitis as it kills many of the competing commensal bacteria that usually keep *C. difficile* under control.

A flare of inflammatory bowel disease can cause acute-onset diarrhoea, however, this patient has no history of inflammatory bowel disease. It is also more likely to cause bloody diarrhoea. Ischaemic colitis occurs due to an interruption in the blood flow to the colon, typically due to a thromboembolic obstruction of the inferior mesenteric artery. It would cause diffuse abdominal pain, shock and bloody diarrhoea. Viral gastroenteritis is a potential differential as outbreaks have been known to wreak havoc on elderly medicine wards. However, the history of recent antibiotic use and the absence of vomiting makes it more likely to be *C. difficile*. Colorectal cancer would usually present with a long history of rectal bleeding and constipation, or it may present acutely with bowel obstruction or perforation.

### 15.  D (Hepatic stellate cells)

Hepatic stellate cells reside within the space of Disse and are the main site of storage of vitamin A. Sinusoidal endothelial cells form a fenestrated endothelium to facilitate the movement of various substances in and out of hepatocytes. Kupffer cells are the resident macrophages of the liver and are found attached to the sinusoidal endothelium. Hepatocytes form 80% of the liver mass and are responsible for many of the liver's core functions including synthesis of various plasma proteins and detoxification. Cholangiocytes line the biliary tree and secrete bicarbonate and water into the bile.

### 16.  D (Glucagon release is inhibited by the paracrine effects of insulin via gap and tight junctions)

The pancreas is primarily composed of acini which secrete enzymes into ducts and are, hence, responsible for the exocrine function of the pancreas.

The islets of Langerhans are groups of cells that are found in between the exocrine components and are responsible for the endocrine function of the pancreas. The alpha cells of the islets of Langerhans produce glucagon in response to hypoglycaemia. On the other hand, hyperglycaemia stimulates the release of insulin from beta cells which promotes the uptake of glucose by cells. As insulin and glucagon have opposite actions, insulin has a paracrine effect on neighbouring alpha cells via gap and tight junctions which suppresses glucagon release.

The majority of the endocrine component of the pancreas consists of beta cells. The GLUT-2 transporter is found on the surface of beta cells and facilitates the transport of glucose into the cells in a non-insulin-dependent manner. This is the mechanism by which the pancreas can detect blood glucose concentration. If blood glucose is high, more glucose will enter the beta cells via GLUT-2, more ATP will be generated, resulting in closure of the ATP-sensitive potassium channel. This depolarises the membrane which subsequently causes the opening of the voltage-gated calcium channels. The ensuing calcium influx promotes the exocytosis of vesicles of insulin.

## 17. E (Metaplasia)

Metaplasia is defined as a change from one adult cell type to another (in this case, squamous to columnar). Barrett's oesophagus is a condition in which patients with a history of gastro-oesophageal reflux undergo metaplastic change within their distal oesophagus. Constant exposure to acid from the stomach results in this compensatory change in the epithelium. This is an important state to identify as it can progress to oesophageal adenocarcinoma.

Dysplasia is defined as cytological changes associated with malignancy (e.g. nuclear irregularities) without abnormal cells breaching the basement membrane. Dysplastic changes can arise from Barrett's oesophagus. Hyperplasia is an increase in cell number. Hypertrophy is an increase in cell size. Anaplasia refers to the loss of structural differentiation within a cell.

## 18. C (Transverse folds)

The rectum has a number of features which differ from the rest of the colon. It has transverse folds that are designed to support the weight of faeces.

Taenia coli are longitudinal bands of muscular tissue which are responsible for the peristaltic movements of the colon. They end at the rectum and become a continuous muscular layer. Haustra are pockets in the lining of the colon that facilitate the reabsorption of water. Diverticuli are outpouchings in the bowel wall that are found in the colon, especially the sigmoid colon. Appendices epiploicae are fat-filled folds of the peritoneum that are seen along the outside of the colon. They are not found in the rectum.

## 19. C (Fatty acids are shuttled into hepatocyte mitochondria by the carnitine shuttle to undergo beta-oxidation)

In the fasted state, the body needs an alternative source of glucose, therefore, hepatic glucose output would increase. This will include a combination of gluconeogenesis and glycogenolysis. Fatty acids released from adipocytes will enter the mitochondria of the hepatocytes via the carnitine shuttle. Within these mitochondria, the fatty acids will undergo beta-oxidation which forms acetyl-CoA. The acetyl-CoA, in turn, will be used in ketogenesis.

Alanine aminotransferase is an enzyme that transfers an amino group from alanine to α-ketoglutarate, thereby producing pyruvate and glutamate. Lactate is converted into pyruvate by lactate dehydrogenase. Leucine is ketogenic, not glucogenic. Glycogen releases glucose-1-phosphate, which is later converted into glucose.

## 20. E (Presence of *H. pylori*)

A carbon-13 urea breath test is a non-invasive method for detecting the presence of *Helicobacter pylori* within the stomach. Urease is an enzyme that is produced by *H. pylori* — it hydrolyses urea into ammonia and carbon dioxide. The carbon dioxide will then be absorbed into the circulation and be excreted in expired air. The carbon-13 urea breath test involves giving patients a sample of urea labelled with an isotope of carbon (carbon-13). Following administration, the breath is tested for presence of carbon-13. A positive result suggests that *H. pylori* is present. A stool antigen test may also be used in the identification of *H. pylori*. *H. pylori* is implicated in peptic ulcer disease because it produces a toxin, CagA, which disrupts tight junctions within the gastric epithelium, leading to a loss of epithelial polarity and promoting inflammation. It can be eradicated using 'triple therapy' which consists of a proton pump inhibitor and two antibiotics.

A hiatus hernia is a condition in which part of the stomach herniates through the oesophageal hiatus. It can cause symptoms of reflux. A bleeding ulcer would cause a high serum urea level due to the digestion of red blood cells within the stomach. NSAID use is implicated in peptic ulcer disease because it interrupts prostaglandin production, which normally has a protective effect on the gastric mucosa. *C. difficile* is a bacterium that can cause profuse watery diarrhoea if it overgrows within the colon. A stool sample should be taken to check for *C. difficile* antigen and toxin.

## 21. B (Trypsin)

The pancreas releases trypsinogen (zymogen) into the duodenum where it encounters enterokinase (produced by the duodenum) which activates it to trypsin. This trypsin is then able to autoactivate more trypsinogen into trypsin. Furthermore, it is important in the conversion of other zymogens into their active form including chymotrypsinogen, proelastase and pro-carboxypeptidase. Lipase is secreted in its active form; however, it requires a co-enzyme (colipase) to function at optimum levels. Colipase is secreted by the pancreas in a zymogen form (procolipase) which also requires activation by trypsin once it has reached the duodenum.

## 22. E (2, 3, 4, 6)

Cirrhosis is a condition in which normal functional liver tissue gets replaced by scar tissue due to chronic damage. This usually occurs due to alcoholic liver disease or viral hepatitis. The progressive scarring of the liver results in an inability of the liver to carry out its normal functions. The liver is a major store of glycogen; therefore, cirrhosis can result in impaired glycogenolysis and hypoglycaemia. It is also the site of albumin production, a major plasma protein which is important in hormone transport and maintaining intravascular volume. A reduction in serum albumin can result in fluid overload. A reduced output of bile from cirrhotic livers can compromise the body's ability to digest fat, manifesting as steatorrhoea. Cirrhosis will also cause reduced clotting factor production, thereby resulting in coagulopathy. A nodular, cirrhotic liver will impede blood flow through the liver, which causes an increase in pressure within the portal circulation (portal hypertension). A reduction in intravascular volume due to hypoalbuminemia-induced fluid extravasation will activate the renin-angiotensin-aldosterone system resulting in secondary hyperaldosteronism and hypokalemia.

### 23. D (Auerbach's plexus)

The enteric nervous system is a network of nerves that is responsible for regulating the movements of the gastrointestinal tract. The enteric nervous system consists of two major plexuses: Meissner's plexus (submucosal) and Auerbach's plexus (myenteric). Auerbach's plexus lies between the circular and longitudinal muscle layers and provides innervation to both. The sacral and lumbar plexuses are parts of the somatic nervous system responsible for the sensory and motor innervation of the lower limbs and perineum.

### 24. D (Squamous cell carcinoma)

There are two main types of oesophageal cancer: squamous cell carcinoma and adenocarcinoma. Squamous cell oesophageal carcinoma typically arises in the middle and lower third of the oesophagus and is associated with heavy smoking and alcohol excess. Adenocarcinoma, on the other hand, arises in the lower third of the oesophagus which is exposed to acid reflux from the stomach. Both would present with progressively worsening dysphagia. Barrett's oesophagus is a metaplastic change in the lining of the lower oesophagus in which it changes from squamous epithelium to columnar epithelium. This can then undergo dysplastic changes and eventually become malignant. Although it is true that the oesophagus has ulcerated in this circumstance, the presence of a discernible mass suggests that there is a malignant process going on. Oesophageal webs may arise in the context of severe iron deficiency anaemia — known as Plummer–Vinson syndrome.

## 25.  D (Transverse colon)

The entire gastrointestinal tract receives its blood supply from three main branches of the aorta. The oesophagus, stomach and proximal duodenum are supplied by the coeliac axis. The superior mesenteric artery is responsible for perfusing the intestines in between the duodenum and two-thirds of the way along the transverse colon (near the splenic flexure). The inferior mesenteric artery, finally, is responsible for the blood supply from two-thirds of the way along the transverse colon to the rectum. The area that lies two-thirds of the way along the transverse colon is referred to as the watershed zone as it lies at the distal points of both the superior and inferior mesenteric artery supplies. It is, therefore, at greatest risk of damage due to ischaemia.

## 26.  C (Stercobilin)

The bilirubin metabolism is important to understand as it can have several clinical implications. Bilirubin is a by-product of red blood cell breakdown. Once released from dying red cells, it will travel to the liver where it gets conjugated with a glucuronic acid group via the action of UDP-glucuronyl transferase, resulting in the production of conjugated bilirubin. The conjugated bilirubin is then excreted via the biliary tree into the duodenum. Once within the gastrointestinal tract, commensal bacteria will act upon the bilirubin to convert it into urobilinogen. This is water-soluble and is partially absorbed into the circulation. It will then be filtered through the kidneys and oxidised into urobilin which gives urine its yellow colour. The urobilinogen that remains within the gastrointestinal tract without getting reabsorbed is referred to as stercobilinogen. This can also undergo oxidation, turning into stercobilin which gives faeces its brown colour.

### 27. B (T6–T9)

Sympathetic preganglionic neurons arise from the thoracic and lumbar spinal cord (thoracolumbar origin). The functions of the gastrointestinal tract are considered parasympathetic (*rest and digest*), so the sympathetic activation would inhibit gastrointestinal activity. Sympathetic preganglionic neurones arising from T6–T9 go on to synapse with postganglionic neurones that innervate the stomach.

### 28. A (Painless)

Two of the main causes of obstructive jaundice are gallstones and pancreatic cancer. They may be clinically distinguished by applying Courvoisier's law which states that painless jaundice in the presence of a palpable gallbladder is unlikely to be due to gallstones (i.e. it is more likely to be due to cancer). Cancer of the head of the pancreas can obstruct the common bile duct or pancreatic duct, resulting in obstructive jaundice. Therefore, it should be investigated promptly with imaging and tumour markers (CA19–9).

Widespread itching, jaundice and pale stools can occur in obstructive jaundice due to gallstones. Weight loss is a non-specific symptom that is associated with malignancy but may be incidental.

### 29. C (Parasympathetic vagal stimulation during the cephalic and gastric phases prompts the secretion of pancreatic enzymes)

Vagal parasympathetic activity during the cephalic and gastric phases of digestion results in increased mobilisation and secretion of pancreatic enzymes into the duodenum.

Secretin has no effect on pancreatic enzyme secretion. It is secreted when acidic substances from the stomach enter the duodenum. It stimulates the release of bicarbonate and water from the ductal cells with the aim of increasing the luminal pH. Cholecystokinin is released from enteroendocrine I cells. Trypsin exerts a negative feedback effect on cholecystokinin release. Secretin is released in response to acidic chyme (low pH).

## 30. D (Calbindin-D)

Enterocytes of the duodenum and ileum absorb calcium ions under the hormonal control of calcitriol (active form of vitamin D) and parathyroid hormone. Calcitriol increases the transcription of calbindin-D proteins, PMCA and TRPV6. Vitamin D-dependent uptake of calcium ions across the apical membrane into the enterocyte is mediated by TRPV6 via facilitated diffusion. Cytoplasmic calcium binding protein, calbindin-D, permits the movement of calcium ions from the apical membrane to the basolateral membrane. Given that calcium is a major intracellular signalling molecule, the swift movement of calcium ions across the cytoplasm is essential to prevent this intracellular calcium from inducing various unwanted signals.

TRPV6 is responsible for the transport of calcium across the apical membrane of the enterocyte. Transcobalamin II transports vitamin B12 from enterocytes to the tissues. Hepcidin regulates the absorption of iron via the gastrointestinal tract. Caeruloplasmin is a copper-carrying protein.

## 31. B (High INR)

The consequences of liver failure can be deduced based on the normal functions of the liver. It is the main site of synthesis of clotting factors, therefore, liver failure results in coagulopathy. This can be identified as raised prothrombin time (PT), activated partial thromboplastin time (APTT) and international normalised ratio (INR) on a coagulation screen.

An inability of the liver to produce albumin and undergo glycogenolysis results in hypoalbuminaemia and hypoglycaemia. The serum ammonia level will be increased in liver failure due to an inability of the liver to metabolise nitrogen-containing compounds being absorbed in the gastrointestinal tract. The ammonia can cross the blood-brain barrier and cause hepatic encephalopathy. Liver failure will also impair the ability of the liver to conjugate bilirubin, thereby resulting in jaundice.

### 32.  C (Neutralising stomach acid)

Bile is produced by hepatocytes and released into the duodenum via the biliary tree. Its main role is the emulsification of fats into smaller droplets which can be more easily absorbed. It is also alkaline, which enables it to neutralise any stomach acid that leaks through the pyloric sphincter. Its role in emulsifying fats also means that bile is important in the absorption of fat-soluble vitamins (A, D, E and K).

### 33.  C (Opioid receptor agonist)

Loperamide is a commonly used anti-diarrhoeal medication that works by stimulating $\mu$ opioid receptors in the myenteric plexus of the gastrointestinal tract. Stimulation of these receptors results in reduced activity of the gastrointestinal smooth muscle, thereby resulting in reduced peristalsis. This, in turn, increases the time that the faecal matter spends within the large intestine, thereby allowing more time for the reabsorption of water.

Stimulation of muscarinic receptors (increased parasympathetic activity) and inhibition of beta-adrenergic receptors (decreased sympathetic activity) can result in diarrhoea. Dopamine antagonists (e.g. domperidone) can increase gastric emptying and, therefore, can also cause diarrhoea. Histamine antagonists (e.g. nizatidine) reduce gastric acid production and are used in the treatment of gastro-oesophageal reflux disease.

### 34.  C (Transferrin)

Ferric iron ($Fe^{3+}$) is converted to ferrous iron ($Fe^{2+}$) before being transported into the enterocyte via the divalent metal transporter (DMT-I). The ferrous iron will then bind to intracellular factors which enable it to be moved towards the basolateral membrane. It then moves across the basolateral membrane via the ferroportin channel. The activity of ferroportin is regulated by hepcidin. Once it has traversed the basolateral membrane, ferrous iron will be converted back to ferric iron by hephaestin. It then binds to apotransferrin (unbound iron transport protein) thereby forming transferrin (bound iron transport protein). Iron can also be stored within the enterocytes by forming a ferritin micelle. Dietary haem is bioavailable and therefore is immediately transported through the apical duodenal membrane into the enterocyte by HCP-I.

### 35. C (Mirizzi syndrome)

Mirizzi syndrome is a term used to describe common hepatic duct obstruction caused by extrinsic compression from a gallstone within the cystic duct or the neck of the gallbladder. It will likely present with right upper quadrant pain and jaundice.

Primary sclerosing cholangitis is an autoimmune condition of unknown aetiology which is characterised by the progressive inflammation and scarring of the bile ducts. This scarring can lead to strictures that obstruct bile flow and cause jaundice. Hydatid cysts may be found in the liver and result from a tapeworm infection. They may compress the biliary tree and cause obstructive jaundice. Cholangiocarcinoma is a cancer of the cells that line the biliary tree. It can cause narrowing resulting in painless jaundice. Biliary atresia is a congenital condition characterised by an abnormal narrowing of the biliary tree. It usually presents with neonatal jaundice and is likely to require surgical intervention.

### 36. C (Paneth cells)

Paneth cells are found at the base of the crypts of Lieberkühn and contain acidophilic granules full of antimicrobial enzymes. These cells are also able to carry out phagocytosis and play an important role in regulating the gut microbiome.

Enteroendocrine cells are found within the intestinal brush border and are responsible for responding to various stimuli and producing hormones that regulate the secretion of various digestive enzymes. Goblet cells are responsible for producing mucus to protect the lining of the intestinal tract. Stem cells are undifferentiated cells that migrate upwards from the crypts to replace the cells lost at the surface. Langerhans cells are dendritic cells that are found within the skin.

## 37. B (Copper)

Wilson's disease is an autosomal recessive condition characterised by an accumulation of copper within various tissues across the body. In particular, it tends to accumulate in the liver, resulting in cirrhosis, and within the brain causing a range of neuropsychiatric manifestations that may mimic Parkinson's disease and dysexecutive syndrome. Copper can also deposit within the iris, giving rise to Kayser-Fleischer rings. Wilson's disease is caused by a deficiency of caeruloplasmin, a copper carrying transport protein, which results in an increase in the levels of free copper within the circulation. Hereditary haemochromatosis is a similar condition in which iron accumulates across the body, however, it is less likely to cause neuropsychiatric manifestations.

## 38. B (Spontaneous bacterial peritonitis)

Spontaneous bacterial peritonitis is an infection of ascitic fluid that typically presents with diffuse abdominal tenderness and a fever. Ascites is the accumulation of fluid within the peritoneal cavity which can occur for a number of reasons, including liver failure, heart failure, renal failure and infection. Any static collection of fluid within the body carries a high risk of becoming infected.

Pyelonephritis is an infection of the kidneys which typically presents with loin pain. Patients may also complain of discomfort when urinating. Cholecystitis is an infection of the gallbladder which usually occurs in the presence of gallstones. It usually causes right upper quadrant pain. Viral hepatitis may be acute or chronic. It is rarely painful. Gastroenteritis is an infection of the intestines which may cause diffuse abdominal pain but is also likely to cause diarrhoea and vomiting.

## 39. A (Rectum)

The most common site of colorectal cancer is the rectum, with prevalence decreasing as you proceed proximally. Cancers of the distal colon and rectum are more likely to present with obstructive symptoms such as constipation and complete bowel obstruction. More proximal cancers (e.g. caecum) are likely to present more insidiously. Rectal bleeding may be present in both scenarios, however, in distal tumours, the blood is more likely to be streaked on the stools whereas in proximal tumours it is more likely to be mixed with the stools.

## 40. B (Intracranial bleed)

Polycystic kidney disease is an inherited condition that can follow an autosomal dominant (more common) or autosomal recessive pattern. It is characterised by the presence of multiple cysts within the kidneys. Cysts can also appear within the liver and pancreas. It may present with haematuria and vague abdominal pain. Polycystic kidney disease is associated with the formation of berry aneurysms within the circle of Willis, and it is associated with hypertension due to activation of the renin-angiotensin system. Therefore, patients with polycystic kidney disease are at increased risk of subarachnoid haemorrhage.

## 41. C (Efferent arteriolar dilation caused by ACE inhibitor)

The movement of fluid from the glomerulus into the Bowman's capsule is driven by hydrostatic pressure. It, therefore, requires a pressure gradient to be created between the afferent arteriole (towards the glomerulus) and the efferent arteriole (away from the glomerulus). ACE inhibitors prevent the activation of angiotensin I to angiotensin II. Angiotensin II is a potent vasoconstrictor that, in the kidneys, constricts the efferent arteriole thereby creating a pressure gradient across the glomerulus that drives fluid into the Bowman's capsule. The use of ACE inhibitors, therefore, would lead to efferent arteriolar dilation and loss of this pressure gradient. This does not usually cause many problems in most people; however, ACE inhibitors should be avoided in patients with renal artery stenosis as their renal blood supply is already constricted. Renal artery stenosis is an important cause of secondary hypertension that should be considered in any young patient presenting with hypertension.

### 42.  C (Inhibits Na-K-Cl triple transporter)

Loop diuretics, such as furosemide and bumetanide, are often used to achieve diuresis in fluid overloaded patients. It works by blocking the Na-K-Cl triple transporter in the ascending limb of the loop of Henle. This results in higher concentrations of sodium remaining within the tubular filtrate and exerting an osmotic potential which results in more water being drawn into the filtrate and excreted in the urine.

### 43.  B (Aldosterone)

Aldosterone is a mineralocorticoid produced by the adrenal cortex. Stimuli for aldosterone release include low blood pressure, low sodium and high potassium. Aldosterone binds to mineralocorticoid receptors within the principal cells of the collecting duct and promotes the reabsorption of sodium by upregulating basolateral Na/K channels and epithelial sodium channels.

Antidiuretic hormone increases water reabsorption by increasing the insertion of aquaporins into the apical membrane of principal cells. Fibroblast growth factor-23 is a phosphate reabsorption inhibitor, predominantly acting on cuboidal epithelium cells of the proximal tubules. Angiotensin II acts via the production of aldosterone to increase sodium reabsorption in the collecting ducts. Adrenaline does not affect sodium reabsorption by principal cells.

### 44.  A (It is freely filtered)

Creatinine is a widely used marker of renal function that allows glomerular filtration rate to be estimated. Creatinine is a by-product of protein metabolism and is produced at a constant rate. It is freely filtered at the glomerulus, which means that, under normal conditions, the concentration of creatinine in the filtrate within the Bowman's capsule will be the same as the concentration in the plasma. It does not undergo extensive absorption or secretion. The rate of creatinine production is dependent on muscle mass which, generally speaking, is fixed, and the rate of excretion is dependent on kidney function. If kidney function is normal, the serum creatinine concentration will remain around 60–100 $\mu$mol/L. If renal function is impaired and less creatinine is being excreted, it will begin to accumulate in the circulation giving rise to a high serum creatinine concentration. Factors that affect creatinine production include muscle mass, age, sex and ethnicity. There are various different formulae that can take into account a number of these factors along with the serum creatinine concentration to produce a more accurate estimate of glomerular filtration.

## 45. C (Loop of Henle)

The loop of Henle is the middle segment of the nephron in which the tubule creates a long loop with descending and ascending limbs. The ascending limb consists of thick and thin parts. The thick ascending limb is the site at which the Na-K-Cl triple transporter is located. It actively transports these ions into the interstitium of the medulla thereby making it hypertonic. This creates a concentration gradient between the filtrate travelling down the thin descending limb and the interstitium, resulting in water moving by osmosis into the interstitium and concentrating the filtrate. It is important to note that the thin component of the loop of Henle is permeable to water but not electrolytes whilst the thick ascending limb is permeable to electrolytes but not water, thereby enabling this system to work efficiently in concentrating urine.

## 46. D (Urinary tract calculus)

A urinary tract calculus is a stone that forms within the urinary tract and can get stuck, resulting in intense, waxing and waning loin to groin pain (ureteric colic). Risk factors for ureteric colic include dehydration and obesity. The stones may be managed conservatively, medically (using $\alpha$-blockers to relax the smooth muscle around the ureter) or surgically to remove the stone.

Nephrotic syndrome is a condition in which large amounts of protein is lost in the urine. The urine dipstick would be positive for protein. Appendicitis would cause acute abdominal pain that is worst in the right iliac fossa. The patient is also likely to be very unwell with a fever. A urinary tract infection tends to present with a burning sensation when urinating and mild lower abdominal pain. The urine dipstick would be positive for leukocytes and nitrites. Prostate cancer usually presents with features of urinary outflow obstruction such as frequency, urgency, nocturia, hesitancy, incomplete emptying and dribbling.

### 47. D (Calcium)

Urinary tract calculi are solid deposits that can get lodged within the urinary tract and cause severe abdominal pain (ureteric colic). The most common type of urinary tract calculus is a calcium oxalate stone. Hypercalcaemia is, therefore, a risk factor for the development of urinary tract calculi.

Gallstones may consist of cholesterol or pigment. Cystine, urate and magnesium ammonium phosphate (struvite) stones are less common than calcium oxalate stones. Patients with high urate levels may also suffer from gout. Urinary tract infection by *Proteus mirabilis* is a risk factor for the formation of struvite stones as the bacterium can alkalise the urine and precipitate the stone.

### 48. C (20%)

The kidneys receive 20% of cardiac output. The brain receives 15%, the gastrointestinal tract receives 25% and the skeletal muscles receive 15%.

### 49. A (Carcinoid tumour)

Carcinoid syndrome is a constellation of symptoms that occur due to excess hormone (mainly serotonin) production by neuroendocrine tumours, primarily found within the gastrointestinal tract. Symptoms include diarrhoea, abdominal pain, shortness of breath, palpitations and facial flushing. Carcinoid tumours of the gastrointestinal tract originate from enterochromaffin cells and are generally slow growing in nature. Whilst the tumour is localised, it may not cause any hormonal symptoms as the excess serotonin produced is metabolised by the liver. Once the tumour spreads to the liver, however, it is able to bypass hepatic metabolism and release excess serotonin into the systemic circulation. Given its slow-growing nature, carcinoid tumours have a good prognosis and are often managed medically with somatostatin analogues (e.g. octreotide).

## 50. B (Submucosa)

A defect in the wall of the stomach must erode beyond the mucosa and, hence, into the submucosa, for it to be classed as an ulcer. Defects that are more superficial are classed as erosions. The layers of the gastric wall are as follows (in order of superficial to deep): mucosa (epithelium, lamina propria, muscularis mucosa), submucosa (consists of connective tissue, blood vessels and nerves), muscularis propria and serosa.

# Endocrinology

## Questions

1. Which arteries directly supply the thyroid gland?

   **A** External carotid arteries
   **B** Internal carotid arteries
   **C** Superior and inferior thyroid arteries
   **D** Anterior and posterior thyroid arteries
   **E** Recurrent laryngeal arteries

2. Which anatomical structure is responsible for secreting transparent lubricating fluid in males?

   **A** Epididymis
   **B** Vas deferens
   **C** Spermatic cord
   **D** Bulbourethral gland
   **E** Seminal vesicles

3. Which of the following is true regarding the synthesis of calcitriol?

   **A** Renal 25-hydroxylase hydroxylates vitamin D2 and D3 into 25-hydroxy-cholecalciferol

    **B** 7-dehydrocholesterol is the initial precursor of vitamin D

    **C** 1$\alpha$-hydroxylase catalyses the hydroxylation of 25-hydroxycholecalciferol into calcitriol within the distal convoluted tubule of the kidney

    **D** UV radiation stimulates the conversion of pre-vitamin D2 into vitamin D2 within the epidermis

    **E** Calcitriol auto-regulates synthesis by decreasing transcription of 25-hydroxylase

4. Which region of the adrenal gland predominantly secretes glucocorticoids?

    **A** Zona glomerulosa
    **B** Zona fasciculata
    **C** Zona reticularis
    **D** Adrenal medulla
    **E** Chromaffin cells

5. What is the mechanism of action of insulin?

    **A** Stimulates glycogenesis, glycolysis, and lipolysis
    **B** Inhibits hepatic hexokinase and reduces phosphorylation of glucose into glucose-6-phosphate
    **C** Stimulates the transcription and translation of GLUT-2 co-transporter proteins within myocytes
    **D** Binds to the insulin receptor alpha subunits and induces a conformational change that activates the tyrosine kinase domains
    **E** Inhibits the activity of lipoprotein lipases within adipocytes

6. Which hormone is <u>not</u> secreted into the primary capillary plexus within the median eminence?

    **A** Dopamine
    **B** Somatostatin
    **C** Gonadotropin-releasing hormone

**D** Thyroid-stimulating hormone

**E** Corticotropin-releasing hormone

7. Which order best describes the process by which thyroid hormone is produced?

    **1.** Pendrin pumps pump iodide from the follicles into the colloid via the apical membrane

    **2.** Coupling of MIT & DIT to form triiodothyronine, with the coupling of two DIT molecules forming tetraiodothyronine (thyroxine)

    **3.** Active transport of iodide by basal membrane iodide pumps

    **4.** Thyroglobulin exocytosed into the colloid

    **5.** TSH binds to TSH cell-surface receptors of follicular cells

    **A** $5 \rightarrow 1 \rightarrow 3 \rightarrow 4 \rightarrow 2$

    **B** $5 \rightarrow 1 \rightarrow 4 \rightarrow 3 \rightarrow 2$

    **C** $5 \rightarrow 3 \rightarrow 4 \rightarrow 2 \rightarrow 1$

    **D** $5 \rightarrow 3 \rightarrow 1 \rightarrow 4 \rightarrow 2$

    **E** $5 \rightarrow 4 \rightarrow 1 \rightarrow 3 \rightarrow 2$

8. Which hormone is secreted by Sertoli cells to prevent the development of fallopian tubes in males?

    **A** Anti-Müllerian hormone

    **B** Activin

    **C** Inhibin

    **D** Androgen-binding protein

    **E** Testosterone

9. Which cells secrete calcitonin?

    **A** Chief cells

    **B** Follicular cells

    **C** Chromaffin cells

    **D** Oxyphil cells

    **E** Parafollicular cells

10. A 10-year-old girl presents to her GP complaining of irregular periods and abnormal growth of facial hair. Upon examination, she has a muscular physique and a dark complexion. An examination of her external genitalia reveals clitoral enlargement.
    What is the most likely diagnosis?

    A  Addison's disease
    B  Classical congenital adrenal hyperplasia
    C  Non-classical congenital adrenal hyperplasia
    D  17-hydroxylase deficiency
    E  Polycystic ovarian syndrome

11. Which of the following hormones inhibit glucagon release from the alpha cells of the islets of Langerhans?

    1. Glucose-dependent insulinotropic peptide
    2. Glucagon-like peptide-1
    3. Somatostatin
    4. Insulin
    5. Amylin

    A  All of the above
    B  2, 3, 4, 5
    C  3, 4, 5
    D  1, 3, 4
    E  2, 3, 4

12. Dopaminergic neurones influence hormone secretion from which type of endocrine cell?

    A  Somatotrophs
    B  Lactotrophs
    C  Thyrotrophs
    D  Gonadotrophs
    E  Corticotrophs

13. Which enzyme is responsible for the activation of iodide within the colloid?

**A** Iodothyronine deiodinase
**B** Thyroid deiodinase
**C** Thyroid iodinase
**D** Thyroid peroxidase
**E** Thyroid activase

14. Which of the following events directly enables the transfer of genetic material into the ovum during fertilisation?

    **A** Removal of a glycoprotein layer, revealing acrosomal receptors
    **B** Motility changes such as whipping movements of the tail
    **C** Acrosin digestion of the zona pellucida
    **D** Acrosin induces motility changes within the sperm cell
    **E** Use of sugar-rich seminal fluid

15. What is the function of fibroblast growth factor-23 (FGF-23)?

    **A** Decreases renal phosphate reabsorption
    **B** Osteoblasts secrete FGF-23 in response to elevated levels of calcitriol
    **C** Stimulates the synthesis of calcitriol
    **D** PTH and FGF-23 increase serum phosphate levels
    **E** Decreases sodium excretion in the urine

16. Which of the following would you least expect to see in a patient with primary hyperaldosteronism?

    **A** Acidosis
    **B** Hypokalaemia
    **C** Hypernatremia
    **D** Hypertension
    **E** Low plasma renin

17. Five asymptomatic patients attend a diabetes clinic for a free consultation.
    Which patient is most likely to be diagnosed with diabetes mellitus?

    **A** Patient 1: Oral glucose tolerance test (9.4 mmol/L)

    **B** Patient 2: HbA1c (56 mmol/mol); fasting glucose (8 mmol/L)

    **C** Patient 3: Random glucose (11.1 mmol/L)

    **D** Patient 4: Postprandial glucose (10.5 mmol/L); glucose positive urine dipstick

    **E** Patient 5: Presence of glucose on urine dipstick; fasting glucose (6.9 mmol/L)

18. Which statement is correct regarding the production and transport of thyroid hormones?

    **A** Plasma albumin is the main mode of iodothyronine transport

    **B** Transthyretin binds to circulating thyroid hormones, with a greater affinity to tetraiodothyronine (T4) than triiodothyronine (T3)

    **C** 80% of circulating T3 arises from direct secretion from the thyroid gland

    **D** T3 has a longer half-life than T4

    **E** T4 is more bioactive than T3

19. Which of the following maternal hormones increase during pregnancy?

    **1.** Adrenocorticotropic hormone

    **2.** Luteinising hormone & follicle-stimulating hormone

    **3.** Iodothyronines

    **4.** Thyroid-stimulating hormone

    **5.** $\beta$-hCG

    **6.** Prolactin

    **A** 1, 2, 4, 6

    **B** 1, 3, 5, 6

    **C** 1, 4, 6

    **D** 2, 4, 5

    **E** 2, 3, 6

20. A patient who has recently undergone a total thyroidectomy for thyroid cancer attends an outpatient follow-up clinic. He is shown to have Chvostek's sign on examination.

Which of the following signs may you also expect to see?

A  Cogwheel rigidity
B  Convulsions, arrhythmias, and tetany
C  Paraesthesia and reduced neuronal excitability
D  Muscle fatigue, abdominal and psychic groans
E  Urinary tract calculi

21. A 44-year-old woman visits her GP complaining of poor sleep and low mood over the past 5 months. In this time, she has also noticed that her periods have become increasingly irregular with her last period being 2 months ago.
What is the most likely diagnosis?

A  Ovarian cancer
B  Prolactinoma
C  Polycystic ovarian syndrome
D  Menopause
E  Premature ovarian insufficiency

22. A 39-year-old woman is referred to the endocrinology clinic by her GP after complaining of frequent urination. Her sleep has been disturbed as she wakes up about 3 times per night to go to the toilet. A series of blood tests are conducted.

Hb1A1c: 33 mmol/mol (<42)
Fasting plasma glucose: 5.4 mmol/L (<5.6)
Na: 152 mmol/L (135–145)

A water deprivation test is conducted.

Urine osmolality: 192 mOSm/kg
Urine osmolality with ddAVP: 500 mOSm/kg

What is the most likely diagnosis?

A  Psychogenic polydipsia
B  Cranial diabetes insipidus

    **C** Nephrogenic diabetes insipidus

    **D** Type I diabetes mellitus

    **E** SIADH

23. By what mechanism do iodothyronines induce gene expression within target cells?

    **A** Iodothyronines are peptide hormones that bind to cell-surface receptors to induce a secondary messenger response

    **B** Iodothyronines directly bind to promoter regions of DNA

    **C** Iodothyronines are membrane-soluble, forming receptor-hormone complexes that bind to T3 response elements (TRE)

    **D** Iodothyronine secondary messengers bind to retinoid X receptors

    **E** Iodothyronine receptor-hormone complexes bind to TREs as heterodimers

24. Which of the following best describes the function of theca cells?

    **A** Secretion of the relaxin

    **B** Section of progesterone

    **C** Convert androgens to oestrogens via the action of aromatase

    **D** Synthesis of androgens in response to luteinising hormone

    **E** Secretion of inhibin

25. Which of the following could cause hypocalcaemia?

    **A** Increased calcitonin secretion

    **B** Bone metastases stimulating increased osteoclast activity

    **C** Squamous cell carcinoma

    **D** Parathyroid gland adenoma

    **E** Excess vitamin D supplements

26. What is the main physiological effect of cortisol?

    **A** Increases hepatic gluconeogenesis and peripheral protein anabolism

**B** Stimulates glycogenolysis and fat lipolysis
**C** Bind with high affinity to mineralocorticoid receptors within the kidney
**D** Promote inflammation
**E** Decreases glomerular filtration rate and renal blood flow

27. Which stage is incorrect in terms of insulin secretion in response to hyperglycaemic conditions?

   **A** Insulin secretion from pancreatic beta-cells of the islets of Langerhans is mainly regulated by facilitated diffusion of glucose via GLUT-2 co-transporters
   **B** Glucose is phosphorylated to glucose-6-phosphate by glucokinase and then metabolised to ATP by glycolysis
   **C** Increase in ATP: ADP ratio induces the opening of cell-surface ATP sensitive K+ channels, leading to cell membrane depolarisation
   **D** Voltage-dependent calcium channels open, facilitating extracellular calcium influx
   **E** The rise in cytosolic calcium triggers the exocytosis of insulin from secretory vesicles

28. Which of the following is <u>not</u> considered an effect of thyroid hormone?

   **A** Stimulates tissue calorigenesis
   **B** Increases protein, carbohydrate, and fat metabolism
   **C** Increases hepatic vitamin A synthesis
   **D** Enhances the rate of gluconeogenesis and glycogenolysis, leading to an elevation in serum glucose
   **E** Increases heart rate by enhancing cardiac $\alpha$-adrenergic activity

29. A 30-year-old woman is being investigated in the fertility clinic after failing to conceive despite having regular intercourse for 2 years. Her periods have been irregular for the past 18 months, but she has

attributed this to previously having the contraceptive implant. She has also gained 10 kg in weight over the preceding 2 years and her acne has got considerably worse.

Given the clinical information, what is the most likely diagnosis?

    A  Premature ovarian failure
    B  Hypogonadotropic hypogonadism
    C  Polycystic ovarian syndrome
    D  Turner syndrome
    E  Kallmann syndrome

30. Which of the following is an effect of calcitriol?

    A  Decrease renal phosphate excretion
    B  Suppress osteoblast activity
    C  Inhibit PTH secretion from the thyroid gland
    D  Decrease hepatic $1\alpha$-hydroxylase activity
    E  Increase osteoclast activity

31. Which of the following is the earliest physical feature of puberty in females?

    A  Thelarche
    B  Voice changes
    C  Menarche
    D  Growth spurt
    E  Pubarche

32. Which of the following responses occur during hypocalcaemic states?

    1. G-protein coupled sensing receptors on chief cells detect low serum calcium, stimulating parathyroid hormone (PTH) production
    2. PTH increases the expression of $1\alpha$-hydroxylase
    3. Decreased phosphate excretion from the kidney
    4. Increased calbindin-D transcription within the gastrointestinal tract

**5.** Osteoclast activity increases, resulting in the demineralisation of calcium hydroxyapatite

**A** All of the above
**B** 2, 3, 4, 5
**C** 1, 2, 4, 5
**D** 1, 3, 4
**E** 2, 4, 5

33. A 7-year-old girl is referred to the developmental paediatrics clinic as she appears to be growing considerably faster than her peers. She is tall for her age and has started to develop breast buds and pubic hair. What is the most likely diagnosis?

**A** Congenital adrenal hyperplasia
**B** Androgen insensitivity syndrome
**C** Polycystic ovarian syndrome
**D** Kallmann syndrome
**E** Klinefelter syndrome

34. Which statements are correct regarding the control of iodothyronine production?

**1.** Parvocellular hypothalamic neurones release a thyrotropin-eleasing hormone into the primary capillary plexus
**2.** Thyrotrophs within the posterior pituitary gland, secrete thyroid-stimulating hormone (TSH)
**3.** Elevated serum T3 & T4 result in a negative feedback effect directly acting on the adenohypophysis to inhibit the secretion of TSH
**4.** Elevated levels of cortisol and oestrogen have a stimulatory effect on iodothyronine production
**5.** Ingestion of large amounts of inorganic iodide leads to the Wolff–Chaikoff effect

**A** All of the above
**B** 2, 3, 4, 5

C 2, 3, 4
D 1, 3, 5
E 1, 3, 4

35. Which statements are correct regarding the juxtaglomerular apparatus?

1. Renin is released in response to decreased renal perfusion pressures within the arterioles
2. The macula densa secretes renin
3. Juxtaglomerular cells are modified smooth muscle cells lining the efferent arterioles
4. Sympathetic stimulation of $\beta_1$ adrenoreceptors on juxtaglomerular cells activates the renin-angiotensin system
5. Vasopressin influences the permeability of the renal collecting duct, increasing water reabsorption

A All of above
B 1, 3, 4, 5
C 2, 3, 5
D 1, 4, 5
E 1, 3, 5

36. A 54-year-old woman has gained 7 kg in weight over the past 6 months. She has also been very tired and increasingly sensitive to the cold. On examination, her skin is dry, rough and pale, she is noted to have a small non-tender goitre. Her vital signs are: RR: 13, HR: 51, $SpO_2$: 99%, BP: 129/85.
Given the most likely diagnosis, which of the following are you least likely to see in this patient?

A Tremor
B Constipation
C Deepening voice
D Depression
E Hair loss

37. A 63-year-old patient is referred to the endocrinology clinic due to increased skin pigmentation across his torso and vitiligo on his hands. The patient also mentions that he has been feeling very fatigued recently and has lost around 5 kg in body weight. His vital signs are: RR: 11, HR: 74, SpO$_2$: 98%, BP: 80/40, Temp: 37.6.
Which of the following pathological changes <u>least</u> likely to feature in this patient?

    **A** Elevated melanocyte-stimulating hormone concentration
    **B** Metabolic acidosis due to insufficient aldosterone and cortisol production
    **C** Decreased corticotropin-releasing hormone levels from the hypothalamus
    **D** Adrenal tuberculosis affecting the zona fasciculata
    **E** Hypoglycemia due to reduced cortisol secretion

38. Which of the following hormones is responsible for milk ejection from the mammary glands?

    **A** Orexin
    **B** Dopamine
    **C** Serotonin
    **D** Oxytocin
    **E** Prolactin

39. Which of the following sets of signs and symptoms would you be most likely to see in a patient with Cushing syndrome?

    **A** Hypertension, proximal myopathy, weight loss
    **B** Centripetal obesity, impaired glucose tolerance, red striae
    **C** Pendulous abdomen, postural hypotension, fat pads
    **D** Depression, osteoporosis, hypoglycemia
    **E** Amenorrhea, diabetes, acidosis

40. A 42-year-old patient has been on high-dose steroids for several months for the treatment of sarcoidosis. He attends a routine clinic appointment and is noted to have a blood pressure of 174/98 mm Hg. His blood tests also reveal hyponatraemia and hyperkalaemia. Saturation of which enzyme results in the manifestations described above?

    A  1α-hydroxylase
    B  17α-hydroxylase
    C  21-hydroxylase
    D  11β-hydroxysteroid dehydrogenase 2
    E  3β-hydroxysteroid dehydrogenase

# Answer

## 1. C (Superior and inferior thyroid arteries)

The thyroid gland is supplied by the superior thyroid artery (branch of the external carotid artery) and inferior thyroid artery (branch of the thyrocervical trunk).

The common carotid artery gives rise to the external and internal carotid arteries which are a major component of the blood supply to the brain and face. The recurrent laryngeal nerve is a branch of the vagus nerve that supplies the intrinsic muscles of the larynx.

## 2. D (Bulbourethral gland)

The bulbourethral glands are located posterolateral to the urethra and slightly inferior to the prostate gland. They produce a transparent lubricating fluid that empties directly into the urethra.

The epididymis is located on the posterior surface of each testicle and it is involved in the storage and transportation of sperm. The vas deferens is a muscular tube that enables the transport of sperm from the epididymis to the urethra. The spermatic cord is a structure containing the vas deferens, testicular artery, pampiniform plexus and lymph vessels. Seminal vesicles produce seminal fluid which provides sperm with a source of energy.

## 3. B (7-dehydrocholesterol is the initial precursor of vitamin D)

Initially, 7-dehydrocholesterol is converted into pre-vitamin D3. Then, exposure to UV radiation stimulates the conversion of pre-vitamin D3 into vitamin D3 within the epidermis. At this stage, vitamin D2 and D3 are still inactive. They then undergo hydroxylation in the liver, catalysed by 25-hydroxylase, leading to the formation of 25-hydroxycholecalciferol. This will then be converted by $1\alpha$-hydroxylase in the proximal convoluted tubule of the kidneys into the active form of vitamin D (1,25-dihydroxycholecalciferol) also known as calcitriol.

25-hydroxylase is found within the liver, not the kidney. The second hydroxylation step of vitamin D primarily occurs within the proximal convoluted tubule. Vitamin D2 (ergocalciferol) is derived from yeast and fungi. Pre-vitamin D3 is located within the epidermis. Calcitriol autoregulation occurs by decreasing the transcription of 1α-hydroxylase.

### 4. B (Zona fasciculata)

The adrenal glands are two triangular endocrine glands located on the superior surface of the kidney. They have an important role in the secretion of several endocrine hormones. Structurally, the adrenal glands are divided into the adrenal cortex and the adrenal medulla, with the former split into specific layers. The zona fasciculata produces and secretes glucocorticoids (cortisol), in addition to relatively small amounts of androgens. The zona glomerulosa produces and secretes mineralocorticoids (aldosterone). The zona reticularis produces and secretes androgens and oestrogens. The adrenal medulla secretes catecholamines — adrenaline (80%) and noradrenaline (20%). Chromaffin cells are the specialised cells that make up the adrenal medulla.

### 5. D (Binds to the insulin receptor alpha subunits and induces a conformational change that activates the tyrosine kinase domains)

The binding action of insulin to insulin receptor alpha subunits induces a conformational change that activates the tyrosine kinase domains. Insulin is released by pancreatic beta cells within the islets of Langerhans in response to hyperglycaemic conditions. Insulin decreases serum glucose concentration by increasing glycogenesis, glycolysis, glucose uptake, protein synthesis and lipogenesis.

Lipolysis is inhibited through the downregulation of lipases within adipocytes. Hepatic hexokinase is activated to phosphorylate glucose into glucose-6-phosphate, facilitating glycolysis. GLUT-2 co-transporter proteins are insulin-independent and are found on hepatocytes. GLUT-4 co-transporter proteins are translated upon insulin-receptor stimulation — these proteins facilitate the uptake of glucose within myocytes. Circulating triglycerides associated with chylomicrons are hydrolysed by the action of lipoprotein lipases into glycerol and non-esterified fatty acids. These undergo esterification reactions to form triglycerides in adipose tissue. Insulin potentiates this activity.

## 6. D (Thyroid-stimulating hormone)

Parvocellular hypothalamic neurons secrete regulatory (inhibitory and stimulatory) hormones into the primary capillary plexus within the median eminence of the pituitary gland. These will then influence the production of hormones by the pituitary gland. TSH is released by thyrotrophs of the anterior pituitary into the systemic circulation. This will then stimulate thyroxine production by the thyroid gland.

Dopamine inhibits prolactin release by lactotrophs. Somatostatin inhibits growth hormone release from somatotrophs. GnRH stimulates the release of LH and FSH from gonadotrophs within the anterior pituitary gland. CRH stimulates the release of adrenocorticotropic hormone from corticotrophs.

## 7. D (5 → 3 → 1 → 4 → 2)

Thyroid stimulating hormone, secreted by thyrotrophs of the anterior pituitary gland, will enter the circulation and bind to TSH receptors on the basal surface of follicular cells setting as sequence of events in motion.

1. Active transport of iodide into follicular cells via sodium-iodide symporter. The iodide pumps are located on the **basal membrane**.
2. Pendrin pumps pump iodide from the follicle into the colloid, via the **apical membrane**.
3. **Thyroglobulin** consists of tyrosine residues, formed within the follicular ribosomes and inserted into secretory vesicles.
4. Thyroglobulin is exocytosed into the follicle lumen and iodinated. Iodide is activated by **thyroid peroxidase**.
5. Iodide binds to tyrosine residues on thyroglobulin forming 3-monoiodothyronine (MIT) and 3,5-diiodothyronine (DIT) upon further iodination.

6. The coupling of MIT & DIT occurs in the colloid to form triiodothyronine (T3), and tetraiodothyronine (T4).

7. T3 and T4 are transported back into the follicular cells, being subjected to proteolytic cleavage of tyrosine residues. This liberates T3 & T4 from thyroglobulin and are subsequently released into circulation from the basal surface of follicular cells.

## 8. A (Anti-Müllerian hormone)

During the development of an embryo, anti-Müllerian hormone (AMH) is secreted to prevent the development of fallopian tubes in males. AMH is also used clinically to gauge fertility in women.

Activin is a hormone produced by the gonads which exerts a positive feedback effect on the anterior pituitary gland, resulting in increased production of gonadotropins. Inhibin is a hormone produced by the gonads which exerts a negative feedback effect on the anterior pituitary, resulting in decreased production of gonadotropins. Androgen-binding protein is a glycoprotein that binds to testosterone and dihydrotestosterone and concentrates them within the seminiferous tubules. Testosterone is an androgen secreted by Leydig cells. It stimulates spermatogenesis and is responsible for the development of male secondary sexual characteristics.

## 9. E (Parafollicular cells)

Parafollicular cells are neuroendocrine cells located within the thyroid gland that are responsible for the secretion of calcitonin.

Chief cells secrete parathyroid hormone (PTH). The follicular cells of the thyroid gland secrete thyroxine. Chromaffin cells of the adrenal medulla secrete adrenaline and noradrenaline. Oxyphil cells are located within the parathyroid gland and can produce PTH-related peptide and calcitriol.

## 10. C (Non-classical congenital adrenal hyperplasia)

This vignette describes a patient with congenital adrenal hyperplasia (CAH). It is caused by a deficiency of 21-hydroxylase which is an essential enzyme in the production of adrenal steroid hormones. It cataly-ses the hydroxylation of progesterone and 17-hydroxyprogesterone into precursors that go on to form aldosterone and cortisol respectively. Therefore, a 21-hydroxylase deficiency will be associated with a reduc-tion in these adrenal hormones. This results in the shunting of precursors down the sex steroid production pathway, resulting in an overproduction of oestrogens and testosterone. Classical CAH describes an absolute lack of 21-hydroxylase, which is typically identified soon after childbirth as the lack of cortisol and aldosterone results in a salt-losing crisis (hyponatraemia, hypotension and dehydration). Female newborns may also have abnormal external genitalia. Non-classical CAH is caused by a partial deficiency of 21-hydroxylase. This tends to be identified at the onset of puberty because, unlike in classical CAH, patients with non-classical CAH will continue to produce minimal amounts of aldosterone and cortisol, thereby preventing a salt-losing crisis. The effects of the extra endogenous sex steroids only become apparent at the onset of puberty — especially in girls who typically appear virilised. Presenting features include a muscular physique, male pattern hair growth and oligomenorrhoea.

Addison's disease (primary hypoaldosteronism) is typically caused by autoimmune damage to the adrenal gland. This presents with skin hyper-pigmentation, hypotension and glucocorticoid deficiency. 17-hydroxylase is an enzyme involved in the production of sex steroids and cortisol within the adrenal cortex. A deficiency in this enzyme would result in a sex ster-oid and cortisol deficit, with an increased production of aldosterone (resulting in hypokalaemia and hypertension). Polycystic ovarian syn-drome is a complex condition, characterised by an excess production of androgens. Patients typically present with menstrual irregularities, weight gain and abnormal hair growth.

## 11. A (All of the above)

Glucagon is released by the alpha-cells of the islets of Langerhans in response to hypoglycaemic conditions with the aim of increasing serum glucose concentration. Insulin exerts an inhibitory paracrine effect on glucagon release.

1. Glucose-dependent insulinotropic peptide is an incretin secreted by enteroendocrine K cells — it enhances insulin secretion.
2. Glucagon-like peptide-1 — behaves as an incretin to reduce blood glucose levels in a glucose-dependent manner by potentiating insulin secretion.
3. Somatostatin is released by pancreatic delta-cells, inhibiting both insulin and glucagon secretion.
4. Glucagon release is inhibited by the paracrine effects of insulin via the gap and tight junctions.
5. Amylin (islet amyloid polypeptide) is co-secreted with insulin; it inhibits glucagon secretion and delays gastric emptying.

## 12. B (Lactotrophs)

Dopaminergic neurones from the arcuate nucleus of the hypothalamus will release dopamine into the primary capillary plexus of the median eminence. This will then inhibit the production of prolactin by the lactotrophs of the anterior pituitary gland.

Somatostatin and growth hormone-releasing hormone influence the release of growth hormone from somatotrophs. Thyrotropin-releasing hormone stimulates the secretion of TSH from thyrotrophs. Gonadotropin-releasing hormone stimulates the release of LH and FSH from gonadotrophs. Corticotropin-releasing hormone stimulates the release of ACTH from corticotrophs.

## 13. D (Thyroid peroxidase)

Thyroid peroxidase catalyses the oxidation of iodide to form active iodine, in the presence of hydrogen peroxide. Iodine binds to the aromatic ring on thyroglobulin tyrosine residues. Iodination of thyroglobulin produces iodothyronines. Tetraiodothyronine (T4) can be deiodinated in the target tissue to produce bioactive triiodothyronine (T3) via the action of iodothyronine deiodinase. Thyroid deiodinases include classes of iodothyronine deiodinases.

## 14. C (Acrosin digestion of the zona pellucida)

Following ejaculation, sperm cells undergo a process called capacitation (functional maturation) as the cells ascend the female genital tract. Changes occur in the sperm cell membrane as the removal of a glycoprotein layer unveils several receptors. Changes to the membrane stimulate changes in the motility of the spermatozoon, such as increased whipping movements. Once the spermatozoon reaches the pellucid zone of the oocyte, it binds and induces the acrosome reaction. The release of the digestive enzymes within the acrosome (e.g. acrosin) leads to the digestion of the zona pellucida and the membrane of the spermatozoon, thereby allowing fusion of the nuclear contents of the spermatozoon with the ovum.

## 15. A (Decreases renal phosphate reabsorption)

Fibroblast growth factor is responsible for the regulation of plasma phosphate concentration. It is secreted by osteocytes in response to calcitriol. Phosphate regulation is achieved through suppressed expression of NPT2 sodium-phosphate cotransporter in the proximal convoluted tubule, thereby decreasing phosphate reabsorption.

Osteocytes secrete FGF-23 in response to elevated levels of calcitriol. FGF-23 has an inhibitory effect on the synthesis of calcitriol. FGF-23 and PTH both inhibit renal phosphate reabsorption, thus decreasing serum phosphate. The reduced expression of NPT2 thus reduces phosphate-sodium co-transport, thereby reducing sodium reabsorption and increasing sodium excretion in the urine.

## 16. A (Acidosis)

Primary hyperaldosteronism (Conn's syndrome) arises due to the excess production of aldosterone from the adrenal glands. This is typically due to adrenal hyperplasia or an adenoma. Aldosterone stimulates hydrogen ion secretion into the distal convoluted tubule and cortical collecting duct.

An increase in aldosterone therefore results in increased excretion of hydrogen ions, leading to metabolic alkalosis.

Aldosterone stimulates potassium excretion in the urine therefore excess aldosterone would cause hypokalaemia. Aldosterone promotes sodium reabsorption in the kidneys, therefore excess aldosterone would cause hypernatraemia. By promoting the reabsorption of sodium in the kidneys, aldosterone also increases the reabsorption of water. Therefore, high aldosterone levels will cause hypertension. Renin is released by the juxta-glomerular cells of the kidney in response to low circulating pressure and low serum sodium. High levels of aldosterone would cause hypertension and hyponatraemia, thereby reducing the production of renin through a negative feedback loop.

**17. B (Patient 2: HbA1c (56 mmol/mol); fasting glucose (8 mmol/L))**

To be diagnosed with diabetes, a patient must present with 2 positive tests (listed below) or 1 positive test with osmotic symptoms.

Thresholds for diagnosis of diabetes mellitus:

- Fasting blood glucose > 7 mmol/L
- Postprandial or random glucose > 11.1 mmol/L
- HbA1c > 48 mmol/mol

The presence of glucose on a urine dipstick may alert you of the possibility of diabetes mellitus, however, it is not diagnostic.

**18. B (Transthyretin binds to circulating thyroid hormones, with a greater affinity to tetraiodothyronine (T4) than triiodothyronine (T3))**

Transthyretin (thyroxine-binding prealbumin) binds to circulating thyroid hormones with a lower affinity than thyroid binding globulin (TBG), therefore dissociating from them more readily, and thus being responsible for immediate delivery of T3 and T4. The biological properties of tran-sthyretin give it a greater affinity for T4 than T3. Iodothyronines are transported in the blood bound to plasma proteins, which minimises the uptake of iodothyronines by non-target tissue.

TBG is the main globulin that transports T3 and T4, and it is responsible for 70–80% of thyroid hormone transport. Plasma albumin is responsible for 10–15%. Eighty percent of circulating T3 arises from the deiodination of T4 by the action of iodothyronine deiodinases within target tissues. T3 is the more biologically active form of thyroid hormone, and it has a shorter half-life than T4. T4 is the major hormone product released from the thyroid gland.

## 19. B (1, 3, 5, 6)

1. ACTH: Placental synthesis and release of corticotropin-releasing hormone results in an increased release of ACTH from the pituitary gland.
2. Gonadotropins (LH and FSH) and pituitary growth hormone decrease during pregnancy as the high levels of oestrogen exert a negative feedback effect.
3. During pregnancy, high levels of β-hCG can have a thyrotropic effect which can result in increased iodothyronine output.
4. The rise in iodothyronine output results in a reduction in thyroid-stimulating hormone due to negative feedback.
5. Beta-human chorionic gonadotropin (β-hCG) is released to prevent the regression of the corpus luteum following fertilisation. This enables the corpus luteum to continue producing progesterone to maintain the lining of the uterus until the placenta is able to take over the role of progesterone production.
6. In pregnancy, the dopaminergic inhibition on lactotrophs is reduced, thereby resulting in an increase in prolactin production.

## 20. B (Convulsions, arrhythmias and tetany)

Patients who have had a total thyroidectomy are at risk of hypoparathyroidism as a result of removal of the parathyroid glands. This will result in hypocalcaemia. A reduction in serum calcium results in increased neuronal excitability. Chvostek's sign is a manifestation of hypocalcaemia in which tapping the facial nerve over the zygomatic arch results in involuntary contraction of the facial muscles. Other manifestations of increased neuronal excitability include tetany, convulsions and muscle spasms. Low serum calcium also results in arrhythmias as cardiac myocytes are dependent on external serum calcium.

Cogwheel rigidity is a feature of Parkinson's disease. Paresthesia is the abnormal sensation of tingling due to pressure stimulation on peripheral nerves. Increased neuronal excitability will subsequently affect peripheral nerve sensitivity. Abdominal and psychic groans are usually associated with hypercalcemia. Urinary tract calculi are more likely to occur in patients with elevated serum calcium concentrations.

## 21. D (Menopause)

Menopause is the permanent cessation of periods due to the loss of ovarian follicular activity. Menopause is said to have occurred once a patient has been amenorrhoeic for 12 consecutive months and this occurs, on average, at the age of 51 years. Due to a decrease in the number of oocytes, the ovarian production of oestradiol and progesterone decreases. This results in reduced negative feedback to the pituitary gland and, hence, an initial increase in FSH and LH levels. Symptoms of menopause include hot flushes, night sweats, menstrual irregularities, reduced libido and low mood. Hormone replacement therapy may be used to manage the symptoms of menopause in some patients.

Ovarian cancer tends to arise in post-menopausal patients and tends to present insidiously with bloating and abdominal discomfort. A prolactinoma is a benign tumour of the anterior pituitary that results in excess production of prolactin. Prolactin inhibits kisspeptin neurones within the hypothalamus, which results in downstream inhibition of the hypo-thalamo-pituitary-gonadal axis. This, in turn, leads to secondary hypogonadism. Polycystic ovarian syndrome is a common disease characterised by the presence of cysts within the ovaries, menstrual irregularities and evidence of hyperandrogenism. Premature ovarian insufficiency is defined as menopause occurring under the age of 40 years. It may be diagnosed by identifying a very elevated FSH level due to loss of negative feedback exerted by oestrogen.

## 22. B (Cranial diabetes insipidus)

This vignette describes a patient presenting with osmotic symptoms (nocturia, polyuria and polydipsia), which may initially point towards a diagnosis of diabetes mellitus. However, the blood tests reveal that the patient is normoglycaemic and hypernatraemic (suggestive of profound dehydration). Patients who are dehydrated with a high urine sodium would be expected to produce small volumes of concentrated urine as their body attempts to reabsorb sufficient water to maintain homeostasis. In this case, however, the patient is producing dilute urine (low osmolality) despite water deprivation, thereby suggesting that the homeostatic mechanism mediated by vasopressin (ADH) is defunct. Loss of function of ADH leading to the production of large volumes of dilute urine is called diabetes insipidus. It can either be caused by a lack of production of ADH from the pituitary gland (cranial) or a lack of response by the kidneys (nephrogenic). In this case, the administration of synthetic ADH (ddAVP) causes a rise in urine osmolality thereby suggesting that the patient's kidneys are still able to respond to ADH, but their pituitary gland is not producing any ADH (i.e. cranial diabetes insipidus).

## 23. C (Iodothyronines are membrane-soluble, forming receptor-hormone complexes that bind to T3 response elements (TRE))

The receptor-hormone complexes bind to repeated sequences of DNA, called T3 response elements (TREs). Interactions with these sequences result in the activation of the target gene. Despite being classified as peptide hormones, iodothyronines are membrane soluble, and thus can directly enter the cell and interact with intracellular receptors, without the need to induce a secondary messenger response. Iodothyronines bind to intracellular receptors, forming a receptor-hormone complex. This behaves as an activated transcription factor that modulates gene expression, rather than directly binding to promoter regions of DNA. Homodimers and monomers bind to TREs, whereas heterodimers bind with retinoid X receptors.

**24. D (Synthesis of androgens in response to luteinising hormone)**

Luteinising hormone (LH) stimulates the synthesis of androgens within theca cells. Overactivity of theca cells is associated with the elevated levels of androgens seen in polycystic ovarian syndrome.

Granulosal lutein cells produce relaxin to support oocyte maturation. Granulosal lutein cells and the corpus luteum produce progesterone to maintain the lining of the uterus in the early stages of pregnancy before the placenta is able to take over this role. Aromatisation is the process by which androgens are converted to oestrogens. This occurs within the gonads and adipose tissue. Inhibin is secreted by granulosa cells and has a negative feedback effect on gonadotropin levels.

**25. A (Increased calcitonin secretion)**

Calcitonin is a hormone produced by the parafollicular C cells of the thyroid gland. It inhibits osteoclast activity in bones and inhibits renal reabsorption of calcium thereby reducing serum calcium levels. It is of modest physiological importance; however, it is used as a tumour marker for medullary thyroid cancer.

Bone metastases stimulate increased osteoclast activity, this induces bone resorption of calcium hydroxyapatite crystals, thereby releasing calcium into the circulation. Squamous cell carcinomas secrete parathyroid hormone (PTH) related peptide, which mimics the action of PTH and stimulates calcitriol synthesis. A parathyroid gland adenoma is responsible for the elevated secretion of PTH into the circulation. PTH is responsible for stimulating osteoclast activity, in addition to upregulating calcitriol synthesis by potentiating the activity of $1\alpha$-hydroxylase in the liver. Activated vitamin D (calcitriol) increases calcium absorption in the gastrointestinal tract and reabsorption within the kidneys. Over-consumption of supplements will therefore result in excess serum calcium due to excessive absorption.

## 26. B (Stimulates glycogenolysis and fat lipolysis)

Cortisol is referred to as a glucocorticoid as its main effect is raising plasma glucose levels. It is released as part of a normal stress response. Cortisol stimulates glycogenolysis and lipolysis in order to increase glucose and, hence, ATP production. Cortisol promotes peripheral protein catabolism in order to liberate glucose.

It is a catabolic hormone, not an anabolic hormone. This effect is responsible for the loss of peripheral muscle mass seen in Cushing's syndrome. Cortisol does have the potential to cause off-target effects on mineralocorticoid receptors. However, the kidneys contain $11\beta$-hydroxysteroid dehydrogenase 2 which converts cortisol into an inactive form called cortisone, thereby minimising its impact on mineralocorticoid receptors. At high levels, however, cortisol can saturate this enzyme and cause mineralocorticoid effects similar to that of aldosterone. Cortisol is anti-inflammatory. It inhibits the production of arachidonic acid, thereby decreasing prostaglandin synthesis. Cortisol increases GFR and renal blood flow through its effects on mineralocorticoid receptor.

## 27. C (Increase in ATP: ADP ratio induces the opening of cell-surface ATP sensitive K+ channels, leading to cell membrane depolarisation)

A rise in serum glucose will lead to an increase in the concentration of glucose within the beta cells of the pancreas. This will, in turn, lead to increased glycolysis which causes a rise in the ATP: ADP ratio. This then induces the closure of ATP-dependent potassium channels. A subsequent reduction in potassium ion efflux leads to membrane depolarisation and the opening of voltage-gated calcium channels. Finally, the influx of calcium through these channels results in insulin exocytosis.

## 28. E (Increases heart rate by enhancing cardiac $\alpha$-adrenergic activity)

Iodothyronines increase the body's sensitivity to adrenergic stimulation, thereby leading to increased stimulation of Gs-linked $\beta_2$ adrenergic receptors in the sinoatrial node. This results in an increase in heart rate and cardiac output.

Iodothyronines increase calorigenesis within tissues (production of heat through the digestion of food) and, therefore, play an important role in thermoregulation. The primary response to iodothyronines within target tissues results in an overall increase in the basal metabolic rate. This results from an increase in both anabolic and catabolic reactions involving proteins, carbohydrates and fat. Iodothyronines stimulate hepatic vitamin A synthesis, using beta-carotene as the main synthetic substrate. A reduction in vitamin A synthesis in hypothyroidism leads to subsequent hyper-beta-carotenemia, manifesting as yellowish discolouration of the skin. To accommodate an increase in the basal metabolic rate, serum glucose levels increase, thus resulting in increased glucose liberation from glycogen stores within the muscle and liver.

### 29.  C (Polycystic ovarian syndrome)

Polycystic ovarian syndrome (PCOS) is a common condition characterised by the presence of multiple cysts within the ovaries, menstrual irregularities and clinical or biochemical features of hyperandrogenism (e.g. weight gain, hirsutism). By interfering with the hormonal balance of the menstrual cycle, PCOS can affect ovulation and, hence, fertility. It is also associated with several metabolic problems such as type II diabetes mellitus.

### 30.  A (Decrease renal phosphate excretion)

Calcitriol (activated vitamin D) is a lipid-soluble vitamin responsible for potentiating the absorption of calcium from the gastrointestinal tract and promoting osteoblast activity to transform calcium into calcium hydroxyapatite crystals within bone. In addition to its effects on calcium homeostasis, calcitriol also increases reabsorption of phosphate in the kidneys. Calcitriol stimulates osteoblast activity, thereby facilitating the storage of calcium ions within the bone as hydroxyapatite crystals. Calcitriol negatively inhibits parathyroid hormone (PTH) secretion from chief cells within the parathyroid gland, thereby creating a negative feed-back loop. 1α-hydroxylase is located within the proximal convoluted tubule of the kidney, not the liver — 25-hydroxylase is found in the liver. Calcitriol promotes osteoblast activity. Osteoclast activity is stimulated by PTH which results in increased bone resorption and liberation of calcium ions into the circulation.

### 31. A (Thelarche)

Thelarche (breast development) is the first stage of puberty in females. This will be followed by other features of puberty such as menarche (beginning of periods), pubarche (development of pubic hair) and a growth spurt. Voice changes are usually more pronounced in male puberty.

### 32. C (1, 2, 4, 5)

Hypocalcaemia is defined as a state of low serum calcium concentration. The following metabolic and hormonal changes will take place in response to hypocalcaemic states.

1. Chief cells detect changes in circulating calcium concentrations and respond by secreting PTH.
2. Renal 1α-hydroxylase controls the rate of calcitriol synthesis, there-fore, upregulating its expression results in increased calcitriol and, hence, increased serum calcium.
3. Decreased renal excretion of phosphate is incorrect. PTH released by the chief cells of the parathyroid gland in response to low cal-cium also results in **increased** phosphate excretion by the kidneys. The effect of PTH on phosphate can be remembered as 'phosphate trashing hormone' (PTH).
4. Increased calcitriol production due to PTH results in increased pro-duction of cytoplasmic calbindin-D, a calcium transport protein within enterocytes. This increases calcium absorption in the intestines.
5. PTH activates osteoclastogenesis by stimulating the release of osteoclast-activating factors from osteoblasts. The demineralisation

process subsequently liberates calcium ions from bone into the circulation.

## 33.  A (Congenital adrenal hyperplasia)

Congenital adrenal hyperplasia is a condition in which a deficiency of an enzyme (most commonly 21-hydroxylase) within the adrenal steroid synthesis pathway results in the production of excess androgens. The adrenal cortex is able to produce three main groups of hormones — glucocorticoids, mineralocorticoids and androgens — and there are enzymes and precursors that link these three pathways. Therefore, a deficiency in 21-hydroxylase can reduce the production of glucocorticoids and mineralocorticoids thereby shunting precursors towards androgen production. A complete deficiency of an enzyme in congenital adrenal hyperplasia will present within the first few days of life as the newborn will be unable to produce any cortisol or aldosterone and, hence, will present with a salt-losing crisis. In partial deficiency, on the other hand, children may appear normal until they grow older and show signs of precocious puberty due to their elevated level of androgens.

Androgen insensitivity syndrome is a condition in which cells are unable to respond to androgens and, hence, impairs the formation of male genitalia. Polycystic ovarian syndrome is a relatively common condition that occurs in women of fertile age and is characterised by the presence of multiple cysts in the ovaries, menstrual irregularities and clinical or biochemical signs of hyperandrogenism. Kallmann syndrome is a form of hypogonadotropic hypogonadism that is caused by a failure of production of gonadotropin-releasing hormone by the hypothalamus. Klinefelter syndrome is an aneuploidy in which patients will have the karyotype 47 XXY. Patients are phenotypically male, and the main features include infertility and muscle weakness.

## 34.  D (1, 3, 5)

1. Thyrotropin-releasing hormone (TRH), released from the parvocellular hypothalamic neurons, enters the primary capillary plexus of the hypophyseal-portal system. TRH exerts a stimulatory effect on

thyrotrophs to release thyroid-stimulating hormone, which will act on TSH-receptors in the thyroid gland.

2. Thyrotrophs are found within the anterior, glandular, component of the pituitary. It contains endocrine cells including lactotrophs, somatotrophs, thyrotrophs, gonadotrophs and corticotrophs which are regulated by hypothalamic hormones. The posterior pituitary gland is formed by neural tissue that is continuous with the hypothalamus. It is responsible for secreting oxytocin and antidiuretic hormone.

3. Iodothyronines (T3 and T4) exert a direct negative feedback effect on the adenohypophysis (anterior pituitary gland), and indirectly on the hypothalamus by inhibiting TSH and TRH secretion respectively.

4. Oestrogen stimulates the thyroid gland to produce thyroglobulin. Glucocorticoids, however, exert an inhibitory effect on thyrotrophs when present in high concentrations.

5. The Wolff–Chaikoff effect is an autoregulatory function in which an excess of iodine inhibits thyroid peroxidase activity and, therefore, reduces iodothyronine production within thyroid follicular cells.

## 35. D (1, 4, 5)

1. A reduction in blood flow in the afferent arteriole is detected by the juxtaglomerular cells which release renin and, hence, activate the renin-angiotensin-aldosterone system. This will eventually result in a rise in blood pressure.

2. Renin is secreted by juxtaglomerular cells. The macula densa resides within the distal convoluted tubule, and is responsible for detecting renal perfusion pressure, as well as changes in sodium concentration.

3. Juxtaglomerular cells are myogenic; however, they line the afferent arteriole.

4. Increased sympathetic activity acting directly on juxtaglomerular cells activates the renin-angiotensin-aldosterone system.

5. Aldosterone increases sodium retention and plasma osmolarity. This establishes an osmotic gradient, which results in the reabsorption of water.

## 36. A (Tremor)

The constellation of symptoms seen in this patient are consistent with hypothyroidism. Hashimoto's thyroiditis is the most common cause of hypothyroidism. It is caused by autoimmune-mediated chronic inflammation of the thyroid gland. A reduction in the output of iodothyronines by the thyroid gland leads to an elevation in TSH, due to the negative feedback system. A reduction in thyroid hormone output results in a reduction in basal metabolic rate and a 'slowing down' of bodily processes. This manifests as tiredness, bradycardia, weight gain, depression and constipation. Both hypo- and hyperthyroidism can cause abnormal hair loss. Tremor is a feature of hyperthyroidism. Excessive thyroid hormone levels result in increased sensitisation of body tissues to adrenergic stimulation.

## 37. C (Decreased corticotropin-releasing hormone levels from the hypothalamus)

This case describes a patient with adrenal insufficiency. It often presents with vague symptoms such as fatigue and weight loss, however, other, more specific, signs include low blood pressure and increased skin pigmentation. Primary adrenal insufficiency (Addison's disease) is usually caused by autoimmune damage to the adrenal gland. It is important to note that patients who have one autoimmune disease are at high risk of developing another (e.g. vitiligo, thyroid disease). A lack of cortisol production leads to an increase in the production of corticotropin-releasing hormone (CRH) from the hypothalamus. This will then trigger an increase in ACTH release from the anterior pituitary gland. Pro-opiomelanocortin is a large precursor for ACTH. In the production of ACTH, α-melanocyte stimulating hormone (α-MSH) is also produced. Therefore, high levels of ACTH (as seen in primary adrenal insufficiency) will be associated with a high α-MSH level. As the name suggests, α-MSH stimulates the production of melanin by melanocytes, therefore, high levels will result in increased skin pigmentation. A reduction in the production of cortisol and aldosterone leads to a reduction in mineralocorticoid activity. This includes reduced secretion of hydrogen ions into the distal convoluted tubule, thereby resulting metabolic acidosis. Due to the negative feedback loop, a low cortisol level due to insufficient production by the adrenal gland will result in increased secretion of CRH from the hypothalamus in an attempt to fix this issue. Tuberculosis is one of the most common causes of adrenal insufficiency worldwide. Cortisol, being a glucocorticoid, will cause an increase in blood glucose levels. A deficiency of cortisol will result in a propensity for hypoglycaemia.

## 38. D (Oxytocin)

Oxytocin is a hormone that is produced by the magnocellular neurones of the hypothalamus and is released by the posterior pituitary gland. It stimulates milk ejection from the mammary glands. It is also important in stimulating uterine contractions during childbirth.

Orexin is produced by the hypothalamus and is responsible for regulating arousal and appetite. Dopamine is a major neurotransmitter that gives rise to many clinical manifestations if deranged. A depletion of dopaminergic neurones in the substantia nigra of the basal ganglia causes Parkinson's disease. Dopamine dysregulation within the mesolimbic and mesocortical systems gives rise to the positive and negative symptoms of schizophrenia. Serotonin is another major neurotransmitter that is thought to be important in mood regulation. Reduced serotonin levels are implicated in the pathophysiology of depression, hence why medications to raise synaptic serotonin concentration (e.g. selective serotonin reuptake inhibitors) are used in the treatment of depression. Prolactin stimulates milk production, not milk ejection.

## 39. B (Centripetal obesity, impaired glucose tolerance, red striae)

Cushing syndrome is a constellation of signs and symptoms that arise due to excess cortisol. There are numerous causes including exogenous steroids, and pituitary and adrenal tumours. Common signs and symptoms include centripetal obesity, weight gain, proximal muscle weakness and thinning of the skin. They are also at increased risk of developing metabolic complications such as diabetes mellitus and hypertension. High cortisol levels are associated with weight gain. Cortisol exhibits intrinsic mineralocorticoid-like activity, therefore, through the activation of the renin-angiotensin-aldosterone system and suppression of vasodilatory systems, it causes a rise in blood pressure. Being a glucocorticoid, cortisol causes an increase in hepatic glucose output and, hence, results in hyperglycaemia. Cortisol exhibits mineralocorticoid-like effects, thereby increasing renal hydrogen ion excretion resulting in alkalosis.

### 40.  D (11β-hydroxysteroid dehydrogenase 2)

11β-hydroxysteroid dehydrogenase 2 is an enzyme found within aldosterone-sensitive tissues (e.g. kidneys) which deactivates cortisol to cortisone (inactive). This prevents unwanted off-target effects of cortisol. This enzyme is particularly important in the kidneys where it prevents unwanted mineralocorticoid receptor stimulation by cortisol. When present in high concentrations, however, cortisol can overwhelm the ability of 11β-hydroxysteroid dehydrogenase 2 to inactivate cortisol, thereby resulting in effects similar to hyperaldosteronism (high blood pressure, hypokalaemia, hypernatraemia).

# Musculoskeletal System and Rheumatology

## Questions

1. Which of the following joint changes is most likely to occur in rheumatoid arthritis?

   **A** Swelling of the entire digit
   **B** Ulnar deviation of the hand
   **C** Tenderness over the first metatarsophalangeal joint
   **D** Distal interphalangeal joint swelling
   **E** Bony spurs at the joint margins

2. Which of the following parts of a sarcomere remain constant in size during contraction?

   **A** I-band & H-zone
   **B** I-band & M-line
   **C** A-band & H-zone
   **D** A-band & M-line
   **E** A-band & Z-line

3. An 82-year-old woman is brought to A&E by ambulance after having a fall. Her left leg is noted to be shortened and externally rotated. A plain X-ray of both hips reveals a transcervical neck of femur fracture.
   Which of the following systems will be used to define the extent of displacement of the fracture?

   A  Garden classification
   B  Salter–Harris classification
   C  Gustilo-Anderson classification
   D  Weber classification
   E  Ann Arbor classification

4. Which statement is correct regarding endochondral ossification?

   A  Endochondral ossification involves osteoblast secretion of osteoid into a trabecular matrix
   B  Blood vessels within the endochondrium deposit osteoblasts to the edges of the bone structure
   C  Primary ossification centre forms due to penetrating capillaries, transporting chondrocytes into the medullary cavity
   D  Endochondral ossification is faster than intramembranous ossification
   E  Endochondral ossification involves chondroblasts that secrete cartilage

5. What type of connective tissue fits the following descriptions?

   1. Contains chondrocytes
   2. Is strong
   3. Has a perichondrium with a nerve supply
   4. Retains its shape

   A  Loose areolar tissue
   B  Reticular tissue
   C  Fibrocartilage

**D** Hyaline cartilage
**E** Elastic cartilage

6. A 62-year-old woman has developed ongoing right knee pain which gets worse when walking. On examination, the joint is stiff with a reduced range of motion. She has a background of type II diabetes mellitus and has a BMI of 34 kg/m².
Which of the following is the most appropriate first step in her management?

**A** Intra-articular steroid injections
**B** Total knee replacement
**C** Weight loss
**D** Viscosupplementation
**E** Opioid analgesia

7. Which of the following statements is correct regarding the activation of muscular contraction and excitation–contraction coupling?

**A** Actin globular heads form cross-bridges with myosin-binding sites
**B** Voltage-sensitive dihydropyridine receptors are mechanically linked to ryanodine receptors
**C** Myosin filaments are pulled towards the centre of the sarcomere
**D** During the power-stroke ATP binds onto the myosin head
**E** Extracellular calcium ions directly bind to troponin C complexes on the actin filaments

8. Which bone cells are located within the Howships lacunae?

**A** Osteocytes
**B** Osteoclasts
**C** Osteogenic cells
**D** Osteoblasts
**E** Chondrocytes

9. Which of the following is more likely to occur in osteoarthritis than rheumatoid arthritis?

   A  Early age of onset
   B  Swelling of the distal interphalangeal joints
   C  Raised erythrocyte sedimentation rate
   D  Extra-articular manifestations
   E  Rapid progression of symptoms

10. Which of the following statements regarding type II muscles fibres is true?

   A  The proportion of type II muscle fibres is low in the elderly
   B  Type II muscle fibres have a lower capillary density than type I muscle fibres
   C  Type II muscle fibres are more mitochondria-rich than type I muscle fibres
   D  Type II muscle fibres are better suited for long-distance running
   E  Type II muscle fibres are smaller than type I muscle fibres

11. A 32-year-old man is rushed into A&E after falling from a third-floor window. He has sustained multiple fractures and is being reviewed by the orthopaedic team.
    Which of the following bones would take the longest time to heal?

   A  Phalanges
   B  Metacarpals
   C  Radius
   D  Femur
   E  Tibia

12. Which of the statements below are true regarding cancellous bone?

   **1.** Cancellous bone predominates within the diaphysis of bone and within the medullary canal

2. Red bone marrow resides within cancellous trabeculae and is the site of hematopoiesis
3. Trabeculae of cancellous bone follow the lines of stress, in accordance with Wolff's law
4. The large surface area of the trabecular matrix is ideal for calcium ion exchange
5. Haversian systems consist of a central canal surrounded by lamellae

A  All of the above
B  1, 2, 4, 5
C  1, 3, 5
D  1, 2, 4
E  2, 3, 4

13. Which term refers to activation of additional motor units in order to increase the contractile strength of a muscle?

A  Recruitment
B  Excitation–contraction coupling
C  Selective innervation
D  Selective denervation
E  Loading

14. What is the most abundant type of collagen found in the reticular fibres of the spleen?

A  Type I
B  Type II
C  Type III
D  Type IV
E  Type IX

15. A 77-year-old man visits his GP with complaints about his hearing. On examination, it is noted that he has a prominent forehead, and his legs appear bowed. He mentions that he has been experiencing some dull bony pain in his legs for a long time.

Given the most likely diagnosis, which blood test results would you expect to be abnormal in this patient?

A  Calcium

B  Parathyroid hormone

C  Vitamin D

D  Alkaline phosphatase

E  Calcitonin

16.  Arrange the following five components in order of size, from smallest to largest.

1. Myofibre
2. Myofibril
3. Myofilament
4. Muscle
5. Fascicle

A  1, 2, 3, 4, 5

B  2, 3, 4, 5, 1

C  3, 2, 1, 5, 4

D  4, 5, 1, 2, 3

E  5, 4, 3, 2, 1

17.  A 63-year-old woman is being seen in the fracture clinic after sustaining a distal radius fracture following a fall. This is her third fracture within the last year. She has a background of polymyalgia rheumatica for which she takes 10 mg prednisolone daily. A DEXA scan is conducted, and her T-score is −2.8.

Which of the following is the most appropriate initial treatment?

A  Increase prednisolone dose

B  Bisphosphonate and vitamin D supplementation

C  Calcium supplements

D  Denosumab

E  Teriparatide

18. Which protein comprises the I-band within the sarcomere?

    **A** Actin
    **B** Myosin
    **C** Troponin
    **D** Tropomyosin
    **E** Collagen

19. Which of the following joints is most stable?

    **A** Ankle
    **B** Elbow
    **C** Knee
    **D** Hip
    **E** Wrist

20. Which enzyme is responsible for breaking down neurotransmitters at neuromuscular junctions and preventing prolonged signal stimulation?

    **A** Tryptophan hydroxylase
    **B** Monoamine oxidase
    **C** Glutamic acid decarboxylase
    **D** Choline acetyltransferase
    **E** Acetylcholinesterase

21. Which of the following types of muscle fibres has the greatest aerobic capacity?

    **A** Slow type
    **B** Fast, fatigue resistant
    **C** Fast, fatigable
    **D** Depends on the size of muscle
    **E** Enthesis

22. Which type of growth is associated with the growth of the epiphyseal plates?

    **A** Interstitial growth
    **B** Endochondral ossification
    **C** Intramembranous ossification
    **D** Appositional growth
    **E** Osteogenesis

23. A person picks up a dumbbell with an outstretched arm and contracts their biceps to pull the dumbbell towards them.
What kind of contraction has occurred in the biceps muscle?

    **A** Isometric
    **B** Concentric
    **C** Eccentric
    **D** Fibrillation
    **E** Fasciculation

24. Intensive marathon training is most likely to cause which of the following changes in muscle fibre type?

    **A** Type IIA to type IIB
    **B** Type IIB to type IIA
    **C** Type I to type IIB
    **D** Type I to type IIA
    **E** Type IIA to type I

25. Which of the following antibodies is most specific for rheumatoid arthritis?

    **A** Anti-nuclear antibody
    **B** Anti-dsDNA antibody
    **C** Anti-cyclic citrullinated peptide antibody
    **D** Anti-centromere antibody
    **E** Rheumatoid factor

# Answers

## 1. B (Ulnar deviation of the hand)

Rheumatoid arthritis is a chronic inflammatory condition characterised by damage to the small joints of the feet and hands. Ulnar deviation is a deformity that may be seen in rheumatoid arthritis — it is caused by inflammation and destruction of the metacarpophalangeal joints.

The inflammation in rheumatoid arthritis is confined to the joints so it would not cause swelling of the entire digit (dactylitis). Tenderness and swelling of the first metatarsophalangeal joint (podagra) is a classical feature of gout. The distal interphalangeal joints tend to be spared in rheumatoid arthritis. Bony spurs (osteophytes) are seen in osteoarthritis.

## 2. D (A-band & M-line)

A sarcomere contains a single dark A-band, with half of the I-band on either end. During contractions, the length of the myofilaments is not altered, however, the fibres slide over each other such that the distance between Z-discs will be reduced.

- **I-band:** Denotes the lighter regions consisting of thin actin filaments that are anchored to Z-discs. The thin filaments extend towards the M-line and into the A-band. The portion of the thin actin filaments that do not overlap with myosin filaments is referred to as the I-band. This will reduce in size during contraction.
- **H-zone:** Denotes the gap between the ends of actin filaments, found at the middle of the A-band. This will reduce in size during contraction.
- **A-band:** Denotes the area of the sarcomere occupied by the thick myosin fibres. The length remains constant.

## 3. A (Garden classification)

Neck of femur fractures are relatively common in the elderly and it can cause a considerable amount of morbidity. They typically occur after a fall which may be of relatively low intensity. Elderly patients have lower bone density and so they are at an increased risk of sustaining a fracture. Neck of femur fractures can be first classified based on the location of the fracture on the femur (subcapital, transcervical, basicervical, intertrochanteric, subtrochanteric) and based on the extent of displacement of the fracture components (using the Garden classification).

The Salter–Harris classification is used in paediatric fractures. It describes fractures based on their relationship with the growth plate. Gustilo-Anderson classification is used for open fractures. Weber classification is used for ankle fractures. Ann Arbor classification is used for staging lymphoma.

## 4. E (Endochondral ossification involves chondroblasts that secrete cartilage)

Endochondral ossification involves bone development through hyaline cartilage replacement. This begins with blood vessels within the perichondrium bringing osteoblasts to the edges of the structure. These osteoblasts deposit osteoid in concentric circles around the diaphysis. The bony edges prevent nutrients from diffusing to the centre containing hyaline cartilage, thereby facilitating chondrocyte death. Blood vessels penetrate into the space that is created and delivers osteoblasts which enlarge the medullary cavity and form a primary ossification centre. The secondary ossification centre will form involving a combination of matrix mineralisation and invading blood vessels. Chondroblasts secrete cartilage which provides a precursor for calcification and bone generation. This mechanism is associated with intramembranous ossification, forming a trabecular matrix. Osteoblasts on the surface of newly formed cancellous bone become the cellular layer of the periosteum.

Cancellous bone aggregates near blood vessels condensing into red-bone marrow. The perichondrium consists of blood vessels, not the endochondrium (avascular). The primary ossification centres form due to periosteal bud invasion, whereby penetrating blood vessels transfer osteogenic cells which become osteoblasts. Endochondral ossification takes longer than intramembranous ossification.

## 5. E (Elastic cartilage)

Elastic cartilage is an avascular structure surrounded by perichondrium. It consists of type II collagen interacting with proteoglycans and elastin.

Loose areolar tissue is the most common form of collagenous connective tissue. It lines organs and provides structural support. It also acts as a reservoir of water and salts. Reticular tissue contains fibres that provide stromal support to lymphoid organs (lymph nodes, stromal cells, red bone marrow and the spleen). The tissue is made up of type III collagen. Fibrocartilage is a tough and dense cartilage containing both type I and type II collagen. Functionally, fibrocartilage behaves as a shock absorber and is involved in the healing process. Chondrocytes are dispersed within the collagen fibre bundles. It does not have a perichondrium. Hyaline cartilage is the weakest type of cartilage.

## 6. C (Weight loss)

This patient's presentation and examination findings are suggestive of osteoarthritis of her right knee. Her obesity has meant that she has had excessive forces acting through her knee over a long period of time causing damage to the cartilage. Conservative measures should always be considered and recommended to patients with any medical condition. In this case, recommending that she attempts to lose some weight through diet and exercise will likely bring her some relief.

Intra-articular steroid injections can provide some symptomatic benefit; however, it would not be a first-line measure. Surgical replacement is considered in severe cases where conservative and medical measures have been insufficient. Viscosupplementation involves injecting a lubricant into the knee joint to reduce pain and swelling. This can also provide symptomatic relief, however, would not be considered first-line. Analgesia is important in managing osteoarthritis; however, opioids would not be considered first-line. Paracetamol and NSAIDs would be more appropriate.

## 7. B (Voltage-sensitive dihydropyridine receptors are mechanically linked to ryanodine receptors)

Muscular contraction is initiated following the propagation of action potentials along the sarcolemma into T-tubules. Dihydropyridine receptors embedded within the sarcolemma become activated and are mechanically linked to ryanodine receptors in the adjacent sarcoplasmic reticulum. The subsequent activation of the ryanodine receptors results in the release of calcium ions from the sarcoplasmic reticulum.

In the presence of calcium ions, troponin dislodges from tropomyosin and exposes myosin-binding sites on the surface of the actin chain. The charged myosin head can then bind to these sites forming a cross-bridge. The myosin head, once bound, will work to pull the actin filament towards the M-line. This movement is called the power stroke. During the power stroke, ADP and phosphate ions are released, resulting in a strong myosin attachment to the actin. Once the power stroke is complete, ATP will bind to the myosin head and is hydrolysed by ATPase into ADP and phosphate. This provides energy to reset the globular head, ready for another power stroke. Stimulation of ryanodine receptors results in calcium release from intracellular stores (sarcoplasmic reticulum).

## 8. B (Osteoclasts)

Osteoclasts are large multinucleated cells responsible for the resorption of bone. These cells occupy minor depressions indented on the bone surface, referred to as Howships lacunae. The lacunae are caused by erosion of bone by osteoclast-derived enzymes. Osteocytes are mature osteoblasts that have been enveloped within the bone matrix. They continue to form bone to an extent, maintaining the strength of the bone matrix. Osteocytes reside within the lacunae.

Osteogenic stem cells are derived from mesenchymal stem cells and can differentiate into osteoblasts and chondroblasts. They are found within the deep layers of the periosteum. Osteoblasts are responsible for the synthesis and mineralisation of osteoid during bone formation and remodeling. They arise from the differentiation of osteogenic cells in the periosteum, the tissue that covers the superficial surface of bone, and in the endosteum. Chondrocytes are concerned with producing extracellular matrix components and maintaining cartilage.

## 9. B (Swelling of the distal interphalangeal joints)

Rheumatoid arthritis is a systemic inflammatory condition characterised by inflammation of the small joints of the hands and feet. Its aetiology is not fully understood; however, it is thought to be related to the generation of anti-cyclic citrullinated peptide antibodies which result in damage to the synovium. Osteoarthritis, on the other hand, is characterised by damage to the cartilage found within joints. There are two main factors that contribute to osteoarthritis: abnormal joint composition (some people may have inherently weaker cartilage) and abnormal joint forces (such as obesity or excessive use in sports). Osteoarthritis tends to mainly affect large weight-bearing joints such as the hips and knees, but it can also affect the joints of the hands. Osteoarthritis is much more likely to affect the distal interphalangeal joints than rheumatoid arthritis. Rheumatoid arthritis tends to onset between 30–50 years of age. Osteoarthritis, on the other hand, is more likely to cause symptoms later in life. Rheumatoid arthritis is a chronic inflammatory condition, so it causes a rise in erythrocyte sedimentation rate. Osteoarthritis is not inflammatory. Rheumatoid arthritis is a systemic inflammatory condition and can cause a multitude of extra-articular manifestations such as pulmonary nodules and uveitis. Osteoarthritis is confined to the joints. Osteoarthritis tends to progress slower than rheumatoid arthritis.

## 10. A (The proportion of type II muscle fibres is low in the elderly)

Type I muscle fibres are typically rich in mitochondria and are associated with endurance (e.g. long-distance running). Type II muscle fibres, on the other hand, are more appropriate for bigger and more powerful movements. They do, however, fatigue easily and can only be used for short spells at a time. Once we pass our physical peak in our mid-20s, the proportion of our muscle which is made up of type II fibres will decrease. As they are primarily concerned with short-term use, they do not rely heavily on aerobic respiration and so do not have as much mitochondria as type I fibres and they have a less extensive capillary network.

## 11. D (Femur)

Fracture healing occurs at different rates in different parts of the body. This is largely dependent on the size of the bone and its vascular supply. Following a fracture, a haematoma will form around the fracture site. It will then become inflamed and begin to lay down a soft fibrovascular callus. Over time, this callus will calcify and remodel to leave the bone repaired. The femur is known to have the longest healing time following a fracture.

## 12. E (2, 3, 4)

Cancellous bone is predominantly found within the epiphysis of the bone, and within the medullary canal. Cancellous bone consists of trabeculae, and bars of bone adjacent to irregular cavities. The matrix consists of red bone marrow and is highly vascularised, thus making it ideal for hematopoiesis. Wolff's law states that bone grows and remodels in response to the forces that are exerted onto it. The trabecular matrix follows lines of stress to strengthen regions of bone that experience the highest stresses. The trabecular matrix provides an ideal surface area for metabolic activity, including the exchange of calcium ions. In contrast with cancellous bone, cortical bone consists of densely arranged osteons (Haversian systems). A single osteon consists of a central canal surrounded by concentric rings of the matrix.

## 13. A (Recruitment)

Recruitment is the process by which the brain activates additional motor units in order to increase the contractile strength within a muscle. Motor units are recruited in order of smallest to largest (slow to fast twitch), governed by the size principle. Slow-twitch units (type I) produce less powerful contractions, thus if the brain determines that more force is required, then recruitment of larger units will proceed, that being fast-fatigue resistant (type IIA), and ultimately, fast-fatigable fibres (type IIB). In addition, as the force required increases, the firing rate simultaneous increases, a process known as rate coding. The brain does not have an ability to innervate or denervate muscle fibres. Loading is a term used to describe the strain applied on a muscle by a load.

## 14. C (Type III)

Type III collagen is a major component of skin, vessel walls and the reticular fibres of the spleen, lung and liver.

Type I collagen is abundantly found within the dermis, tendons, ligaments and bone. Type II collagen is abundantly found in cartilage, vitreous humour and the nucleus pulposus of the intervertebral discs. Type IV collagen forms the basal lamina. Type IX collagen is another component of cartilage.

## 15. D (Alkaline phosphatase)

This patient has presented with symptoms suggestive of Paget's disease of the bone. It is a relatively common condition that predominantly affects elderly patients and is characterised by increased bone turnover, usually affecting the skull. Most patients will be asymptomatic; however, it can cause bone pain and hearing issues if the disease affects the inner ear. It can also cause bone deformities such as bowed legs. Despite resulting from increased bone turnover, it does not cause any abnormalities in calcium metabolism. It would, however, be associated with a markedly increased alkaline phosphatase which is a marker of bone turnover that is produced by osteoblasts.

## 16. C (3, 2, 1, 5, 4)

Myofilaments are the light and dark bands within a sarcomere, composed of actin and myosin respectively. Myofibrils are 1–2 μm in size and, unlike myofilaments, myofibrils extend along the entire length of myofibres. Myofibres are individual muscle cells that are encapsulated by sarcolemma. T-tubules penetrate into the centre of the skeletal muscle cells providing a conduit for action potential propagation. Myofibres are arranged in bundles (fascicles) surrounded by an intermediate layer of connective tissue called the perimysium. The fascicular arrangement enables the system to trigger specific movement of a muscle by activating a subset of muscle fibres within a fascicle of the muscle. Lastly, a group of fascicles collectively form a muscle.

### 17. B (Bisphosphonates and vitamin D supplementation)

Osteoporosis is a condition in which patients have reduced bone mineral density. A DEXA scan is used to assess bone mineral density, and it gives the value as a 'T-score'. This number quantifies the difference in bone mineral density between the patient and a young, healthy control. Osteoporosis is defined as a T-score of less than –2.5. Major risk factors for osteoporosis include age, menopause and long-term steroid use. Bisphosphonates are the first-line agents used to treat osteoporosis. They reduce osteoclast activity and get deposited in bone thereby improving bone mineral density. Patients will also be started on vitamin D and calcium supplements as this will improve their bone mineralisation.

Increasing the dose of prednisolone would worsen this patient's osteoporosis. Calcium supplements alone would not be sufficient to improve this patient's bone mineral density and reduce their risk of fractures. Denosumab is a RANK ligand inhibitor which prevents the activation of osteoclasts. It is used as a second-line treatment for osteoporosis. Teriparatide is a parathyroid hormone analogue that may be used by specialists in some patients with osteoporosis.

### 18. A (Actin)

The I-bands are lighter regions containing thin actin filaments anchored to the Z-discs. These thin filaments extend into the A-band towards the M-line. There are no myosin overlapping filaments in the I-band.

Myosin forms the thicker filaments which are found within the A band. Troponin and tropomyosin are protein complexes that are found on the surface of actin filaments. Each myofibre is encased by a thin layer of collagen and reticular fibres, forming the endomysium.

## 19. D (Hip)

There is an inverse relationship between joint mobility and stability. Poor stability of joints contributes to an increased risk of dislocation. The hip joint is a deep ball and socket joint surrounded by a strong capsule and reinforced by three extracapsular ligaments. It is also surrounded by several powerful muscles which makes the joint incredibly stable.

## 20. E (Acetylcholinesterase)

Upon the arrival of an action potential at the presynaptic membrane of the neuromuscular junction, acetylcholine (ACh) is exocytosed into the synaptic cleft. ACh diffuses across the synapse and binds to postsynaptic ACh receptors within the motor-end plate of the sarcolemma. Acetylcholinesterases then hydrolyse the ACh within the synapse to prevent prolonged signal stimulation.

Tryptophan hydroxylases are located within serotonergic synapses. It is the rate-limiting enzyme in serotonin synthesis, and it is responsible for catalysing the production of 5-hydroxytryptophan. Monoamine oxidases are responsible for the degradation of monoamine neurotransmitters (dopamine, serotonin and noradrenaline). Glutamic acid decarboxylase is an enzyme that decarboxylates glutamate to form GABA at GABAergic synapses. GABA is one of the main inhibitory neurotransmitters found within the brain. Choline acetyltransferase is an enzyme involved in synthesising ACh in the cytoplasm of the axon terminal.

## 21. A (Slow type)

Type I fibres are slow type oxidative fibres associated with producing sustained contractions. They are responsible for maintaining posture and stabilising joints. These fibres have a high concentration of mitochondria, which means that they have a high capacity for oxidative phosphorylation and the synthesis of ATP. This enables the fibres to sustain a contraction for long periods of time.

Type II (fast) fibres are divided into two subtypes: Type IIA (fatigue-resistant), and type IIB (fatigable). Type IIA fibres are also heavily reliant on aerobic respiration and have a high capacity for ATP production. Type IIB fibres mainly generate ATP through anaerobic respiration which produces less ATP per cycle, therefore they fatigue faster. The reliance on anaerobic respiration, however, does allow the short, forceful contractions. The size of the muscle has no impact on aerobic capacity. This is primarily dictated by the concentration of mitochondria.

**22.  A (Interstitial growth)**

Epiphyseal plates (also known as growth plates) are cartilaginous areas found in between the epiphysis and the diaphysis. The epiphyseal plate is divided into zones. The reserve zone is closest to the epiphyseal end of the plate and contains chondrocytes. It secures the epiphyseal plate to the overlying osseous tissue of the epiphysis. The proliferative zone contains large chondrocytes that undergo cell division to replace the cells that are dying at the diaphyseal side of the plate. The zone of maturation and hypertrophy consists of mature cells and is the site at which longitudinal bone growth takes place. The zone of calcification is found closest to the diaphysis and is the site at which capillaries from the diaphysis penetrate this cartilage and deliver osteoblasts to ossify the tissue.

Endochondral ossification is a type of bone production in which bone is constructed upon a hyaline cartilage scaffold. Intramembranous ossification is a form of bone formation involving mesenchymal cells that undergo differentiation into osteogenic cells. It forms flat bones. Appositional growth refers to the deposition of bone beneath the periosteum to increase the diameter of the bone. Osteogenesis refers to the process of bone development and formation.

## 23. B (Concentric)

Concentric movement occurs when the muscle length shortens in order to shift a load, since the force generated by the muscles sufficiently overcomes that of the load.

In isometric contractions, the muscle length remains constant despite the generation of tension. Lifting shopping bags with outstretched arms is a form of isometric contraction. An eccentric contraction is when the muscle lengthens whilst remaining under tension. Lowering the dumbbell during a bicep curl is a form of eccentric contraction. A fibrillation is an abnormal contraction in a single muscle fibre. It is not visible to the naked eye. It is associated with lower motor neurone disease. A fasciculation is a visible, abnormal twitch in a muscle. It is also associated with lower motor neurone disease.

## 24. B (Type IIB to type IIA)

Endurance training (e.g. marathons) requires the development of fatigue-resistant muscle fibres. Therefore, the most likely conversion in muscle fibre type would be from type IIB (fatigable) to type IIA (fatigue-resistant). Type IIA fibres have a greater capacity for aerobic respiration and, hence, can sustain contractions for a longer period of time.

## 25. C (Anti-cyclic citrullinated peptide antibody)

Rheumatoid arthritis is a systemic inflammatory condition that is characterised by the inflammation of multiple small joints, usually in the hands and feet. Anti-cyclic citrullinated peptide antibodies are highly specific for rheumatoid arthritis and are present in the majority of patients who have the disease. Although the pathogenesis of rheumatoid arthritis has not been fully resolved, it is thought to be related to aberrant citrullination of proteins within the synovium. These proteins are then mistakenly identified as foreign by the immune system, resulting in the generation of anti-cyclic citrullinated peptide antibodies.

# Dermatology

## Questions

1. Which cells are direct derivatives of melanoblasts?

   **A** Differentiated melanocytes and neural crest cells
   **B** Neural crest cell and transit-amplifying cells
   **C** Melanocyte stem cells and differentiated melanocytes
   **D** Differentiated melanocytes and transit-amplifying cells
   **E** Melanocyte stem cells and neural crest cells

2. An 18-year-old man has presented to his GP with a rash that has developed over the past week. Multiple scaly plaques are seen across his torso. He has recently been treated with a course of antibiotics for tonsillitis.
   What is the most likely diagnosis?

   **A** Atopic eczema
   **B** Seborrhoeic dermatitis
   **C** Seborrhoeic keratosis
   **D** Guttate psoriasis
   **E** Drug reaction

3. Which of the following groups of molecules are the major constituents of the basement membrane?

   **1.** Collagen type IV
   **2.** Collagen type V
   **3.** Glycoprotein
   **4.** Integrins
   **5.** Merkel cells
   **6.** Langerhans cells

   **A** 1, 6, 2
   **B** 3, 4, 5
   **C** 1, 3, 4
   **D** 2, 6, 4
   **E** 6, 5, 2

4. Which of the following statements is correct regarding the structure of the dermis?

   **A** The reticular layer is a superficial layer that acts as an anchor point for the epidermis
   **B** The reticular layer is composed of loose, areolar tissue
   **C** Meissner corpuscles reside within the reticular layer
   **D** Type I & III collagen, elastin, and fibrillin are the main proteins that form the dermis
   **E** The papillary layer projects into the stratum corneum as dermal papillae

5. Which of the following describes the correct sequence of skin development?

   **1.** Formation of vernix caseosa
   **2.** Ventral migration of melanocytes to developing epidermis
   **3.** Lanugo hair emerges
   **4.** The epidermis forms as a single layer of cuboidal cells
   **5.** Hair follicles develop from the stratum spinosum

**6.** Development of epidermal layers, the stratum spinosum being the most superficial layer

**A** 4→ 1→ 3
**B** 6→ 5→ 3
**C** 4→ 5→ 2
**D** 6→ 1→ 3
**E** 2→ 1→ 5

6. Which statement describing thermoregulation by sweat glands is correct?

**A** Eccrine sweat glands produce hypertonic sweat for thermoregulation
**B** Apocrine glands are primarily located on the palms and soles
**C** Eccrine glands release sweat through merocrine secretion
**D** Apocrine glands respond to both adrenergic and cholinergic innervation
**E** Apocrine glands are the primary components of thermoregulation

7. Which statement describing the structure of the pilosebaceous unit is correct?

**A** The isthmus is the uppermost portion of the hair follicle
**B** Hair follicle stem cells reside within the bulge
**C** The cortex forms the central core of the hair shaft and root
**D** The arrector pili muscles relax in response to sympathetic stimulation
**E** The infundibulum is the region between the opening of the sebaceous gland and the insertion of the arrector pili muscle

8. Which of the following describes the correct sequence of phases of the hair cycle?

**A** Catagen, telogen, anagen
**B** Telogen, catagen, anagen

    **C** Telogen, anagen, catagen

    **D** Anagen, catagen, telogen

    **E** Anagen, telogen, catagen

9. An 8-year-old boy drops a toy that he was gripping between his fingertips.
   Which nerve ending transducer is primarily involved in detecting the dropped toy?

    **A** Meissner corpuscle

    **B** Ruffini corpuscle

    **C** Pacinian corpuscle

    **D** Merkel cells

    **E** Free nerve endings

10. A 27-year-old man has presented to the dermatology clinic with worsening plaque psoriasis. He has tried emollients and a course of potent topical corticosteroids, but his condition has not improved. Which of the following is a treatment that may be used in his case?

    **A** Radiofrequency ablation

    **B** Ultraviolet light

    **C** Shockwave lithotripsy

    **D** Radiotherapy

    **E** Transcutaneous electrical nerve stimulation

11. Which epidermal layer consists of protruding cell processes that connect cells via desmosomes?

    **A** Stratum corneum

    **B** Stratum lucidum

    **C** Stratum granulosum

    **D** Stratum spinosum

    **E** Stratum basale

12. A 37-year-old patient with a background of plaque psoriasis is undergoing UVA treatment. He has recently developed changes in his fingernails.
Which of the following changes is most likely to be seen?

    **A** Splinter haemorrhages
    **B** Tar staining
    **C** Paronychia
    **D** Koilonychia
    **E** Subungual hyperkeratosis

13. An 81-year-old man presents to his GP after noticing a strange spot on the side of his nose. On examination, there is a 1 cm by 1 cm spot with a raised edge and prominent capillaries around the outside. What is the most likely diagnosis?

    **A** Melanoma
    **B** Basal cell carcinoma
    **C** Squamous carcinoma
    **D** Keratoacanthoma
    **E** Actinic keratosis

14. A 20-year-old man develops streaks of red, raised blisters on his shins a day after walking through a bush of poison ivy.
What is the most likely diagnosis?

    **A** Atopic dermatitis
    **B** Seborrhoeic dermatitis
    **C** Allergic contact dermatitis
    **D** Irritant contact dermatitis
    **E** Venous eczema

15. An 81-year-old woman has been referred to the dermatology clinic after developing tense blisters across her legs. They have been causing her a considerable degree of discomfort and some of them have

burst. A skin biopsy is sent for immunofluorescence analysis which reveals deposition of IgG across the basement membrane.
What is the most likely diagnosis?

A  Pemphigus vulgaris
B  Pemphigus foliaceus
C  Bullous pemphigoid
D  Erythema multiforme
E  Bullous impetigo

# Answers

## 1. C (Melanocyte stem cells and differentiated melanocytes)

There are two main steps in the development of mature melanocytes. Firstly, embryonic neural crest cells give rise to a diverse array of pluripotent cells, including melanoblasts. These melanoblasts then differentiate into either fully differentiated melanocytes or melanocyte stem cells.

## 2. D (Guttate psoriasis)

Psoriasis is a chronic inflammatory skin condition characterised by the development of scaly plaques. There are several types of psoriasis that are described based on the pattern of the rash. Guttate psoriasis has a 'raindrop' appearance as it causes a large number of small plaques. It classically arises after a streptococcal throat infection.

Atopic eczema is a common skin condition characterised by the development of dry, itchy skin, particularly in the flexures. It usually presents in childhood and is often associated with hay fever, asthma and food allergy. Seborrhoeic dermatitis is a benign skin condition caused by *Malassezia*. It appears as a scaly rash on the face and scalp. Seborrhoeic keratosis is a benign skin condition seen mainly in elderly patients. The lesions are usually pigmented and have a 'stuck on' appearance. The use of amoxicillin or ampicillin in the treatment of upper respiratory tract infections must be done with caution. Glandular fever (caused by EBV) has a similar presentation to streptococcal throat infections, however, the use of amoxicillin or ampicillin in glandular fever causes a generalised rash.

## 3. C (1, 3, 4)

Collagen type IV, glycoprotein and integrins are major components of the basement membrane.

Collagen type V is found only in small quantities in the basement membrane. Merkel cells are responsible for light touch sensation and are found within the stratum basale of the epidermis. Langerhans cells are the resident dendritic cells of the skin.

**4. D (Type I & III collagen, elastin, and fibrillin are the main proteins that form the dermis)**

The dermis consists of two layers of connective tissue that are composed of an interconnected mesh of elastin and collagen fibres produced by fibroblasts. The papillary layer is the superficial layer that acts as an anchor point for the epidermis by projecting into the stratum basale via dermal papillae. It consists of loose, areolar connective tissues. Meissner corpuscles are found within the papillary layer — they are mechanoreceptors that are responsible for light touch sensation. The reticular layer lies deep to the papillary layer and makes up most of the dermis. It consists of dense, irregular connective tissue that gives the dermis its multilateral force resistant properties.

**5. A (4 → 1 → 3)**

*In utero*, the skin development will begin at around week 4 when the epidermis forms as a single layer of cuboidal cells. Then a secondary layer of squamous, non-keratinising cuboidal cells (periderm) will develop, resulting in the formation of the vernix caseosa. Melanocytes then migrate dorsally to the developing epidermis and hair follicles. Hair follicles will then continue development in the stratum germinativum, resulting in the formation of lanugo hair.

**6. C (Eccrine glands release sweat through merocrine secretion)**

Sweat is an essential component of thermoregulation. The evaporation of sweat transfers heats away from the body, creating a cooling effect. There are two main types of sweat glands: eccrine and apocrine. Eccrine glands produce hypotonic sweat, meaning that the sweat contains a lower electrolyte concentration than the sweat produced by apocrine glands. They have a coiled tubular structure that releases sweat via exocytosis into ducts that lead directly to the surface of the skin — this is referred to as merocrine secretion. They can respond to both adrenergic and cholinergic stimulation. Eccrine glands are found in abundance in the palms and soles. Apocrine glands are primarily found in the axilla, groin and around the nipples. They also have a coiled, tubular structure; however, they secrete sweat into ducts that lead to hair follicles. Apocrine glands can only respond to adrenergic stimulation and they are thought to be the main contributor to body odour.

### 7. B (Hair follicle stem cells reside within the bulge)

The pilosebaceous unit is a structural unit consisting of the hair shaft, hair follicle, arrector pili muscle and the sebaceous gland. Hair follicle stem cells are found within the hair bulge.

The isthmus is the inferior region of the hair follicle. The medulla forms the central core of the hair shaft and root. The cortex is the layer of compressed, keratinised cells lying superficial to the medulla. The arrector pili muscles contract in response to sympathetic stimulation to stand the hair shafts on end. This traps a layer of insulated air and contributes to thermoregulation. The infundibulum is the superior region of the hair follicle which defines the opening of the sebaceous gland to the surface of the skin.

### 8. D (Anagen, catagen, telogen)

The hair cycle consists of three phases.

1. **Anagen:** The active growth phase lasting 2–7 years. Cells within the bulb rapidly divide, adding to the hair shaft.
2. **Catagen:** The transition phase that demarcates the end of active hair growth, when the hair becomes detached from the blood supply. This lasts 2–3 weeks.
3. **Telogen:** The resting phase during which there is no new growth, lasting 3–4 months.

### 9. B (Ruffini corpuscle)

There are four types of encapsulated mechanoreceptors within the skin: Meissner corpuscles, Ruffini corpuscles, Pacinian corpuscles and

Merkel cells. Ruffini corpuscles are found deep within the dermis and respond to stretching of the skin. They provide feedback for gripping objects and are found at high-density at the fingertips.

Meissner corpuscles are located in the upper dermis and respond to fine touch and low-frequency vibration. Pacinian corpuscles are located deep in the dermis and respond to deep pressure and high-frequency vibration. Merkel cells are located in the stratum basale of the epidermis and respond to light touch, allowing location of a stimulus to be pinpointed. Free nerve endings are non-encapsulated and respond to noxious and thermal stimuli.

## 10.  B (Ultraviolet light)

Psoriasis is a chronic inflammatory skin condition that results in the appearance of scaly plaques across the body. The mainstay of treatment involves topical agents (emollients, corticosteroids and vitamin D analogues). If topical therapies are ineffective, patients may be considered for UV light therapy. Other options include immunosuppressants, such as methotrexate and ciclosporin, and biological agents.

Radiofrequency ablation is a technique used in cardiology to seal aberrant electrical pathways that can lead to arrhythmias. Shockwave lithotripsy is a technique used in urology to non-invasively breakdown a urinary tract calculus. Radiotherapy is the use of high-energy particles or waves to kill cancer cells. Transcutaneous electrical nerve stimulation is a non-invasive method of helping manage pain.

## 11.  D (Stratum spinosum)

The epidermis is composed of keratinised, stratified squamous epithelium and has four or five layers (depending on the location within the body). The layers from superficial to deep can be remembered using the mnemonic *Come let's get sun burnt* which stands for corneum, lucidum, granulosum, spinosum and basale. The stratum spinosum contains keratinocytes with protruding cell processes that join the cells via desmosomes. The desmosomes interlock and strengthen bonds between the cells.

The stratum corneum is the most superficial layer of the epidermis. Thick keratinisation of the cells creates a semipermeable barrier that prevents the penetration of external microbes and prevents excessive fluid loss. The stratum lucidum only exists in the thick skin of the palms and soles. It consists of flat cells containing lipids which gives it a waterproof quality. The stratum granulosum has a grainy appearance as the keratinocytes change as they are pushed from the stratum spinosum. They become flatter and generate large amounts of keratin. The stratum basale is the deepest epidermal layer that attaches the epidermis to the basal lamina.

### 12. E (Subungual hyperkeratosis)

Psoriasis can also lead to changes in the fingernails. There are three main changes that are associated with psoriasis: onycholysis (separation of the nail plate from the nail bed), pitting and subungual hyperkeratosis.

Splinter haemorrhages are dark lines that are seen in the nail and they are classically associated with infective endocarditis. Tar staining is seen on the fingernails of heavy smokers. Paronychia is a superficial skin infection located at the edges of a nail. The area will appear swollen and tender. Koilonychia is spooning of the nails and it is usually associated with severe iron deficiency anaemia.

### 13. B (Basal cell carcinoma)

Basal cell carcinoma is a relatively common type of skin, especially in elderly Caucasian people. It is a slow-growing cancer that does not tend to metastasise and is usually described as having a raised, 'pearly' appearance with a rolled edge and surrounding telangiectasia.

Melanoma is a malignancy of the melanocytes. It is the most aggressive type of skin cancer as it has an ability to spread rapidly. Squamous cell carcinoma tends to appear as a firm lump with a rough surface that may be ulcerated. Keratoacanthoma is a benign tumour that has a similar appearance to squamous cell carcinoma. Actinic keratosis is a rough, scaly patch of skin that arises in sun-exposed areas due to long-term exposure to sunlight.

## 14.  C (Allergic contact dermatitis)

Allergic contact dermatitis is a delayed type IV hypersensitivity reaction that results in inflammation of the skin within the days following contact with an allergen.

Atopic dermatitis (eczema) is a common condition characterised by very dry and itchy skin. Seborrhoeic dermatitis is a common skin condition caused by *Malassezia* that manifests as scaly patches on the scalp and face. Irritant contact dermatitis is a non-immunological inflammatory reaction that occurs due to the direct toxic effects of a particular irritant. Venous eczema arises in patients with chronic venous insufficiency.

## 15.  C (Bullous pemphigoid)

Bullous pemphigoid is an autoimmune blistering disease that is characterised by the formation of large, tense bullae that may rupture. It is caused by IgG antibodies that are directed against components of hemidesmosomes found at the basement membrane. The ensuing autoimmune attack results in a separation of the epidermis from the dermis.

Pemphigus vulgaris is another autoimmune blistering condition that is caused by autoantibody-mediated attack of the epidermis. It results in separation of the upper epidermis from the lower epidermis, therefore the blisters in pemphigus vulgaris are more flaccid than in bullous pemphigoid. Pemphigus foliaceus is caused by autoimmune damage to the uppermost layers of the epidermis. It gives rise to very flaccid blisters that are extremely prone to rupturing such that it is rare to see intact blisters. Erythema multiforme is a hypersensitivity reaction that is usually triggered by infections and gives rise to target-shaped macules. Bullous impetigo is a skin infection, caused by *Staphylococcus aureus*, that forms large, tense blisters. It is more common in children.

# Mock Exam

## Questions

1. A 76-year-old man with a background of COPD, is brought into A&E with worsening shortness of breath and a productive cough. On admission, he has a temperature of 38.1°C, SaO$_2$ of 85% on room air and a respiratory rate of 28 breaths/min. He is started on 4 L/min of oxygen via a nasal cannula and a chest X-ray reveals dense consolidation in the left lower lobe consistent with community-acquired pneumonia.
   Which of the following is the most common cause of community-acquired pneumonia?

   A  *Klebsiella pneumoniae*
   B  *Chlamydia pneumoniae*
   C  *Mycoplasma pneumoniae*
   D  *Streptococcus pneumoniae*
   E  *Staphylococcus aureus*

2. Congenital leptin deficiency is a genetic condition caused by a mutation in the LEP gene. It results in severe obesity.
   What is the underlying pathophysiological mechanism by which leptin deficiency causes obesity?

    **A** Stimulation of anorexigenic neurons of the ventromedial nucleus

    **B** Stimulation of orexigenic neurons of the lateral hypothalamic area

    **C** Stimulation of POMC neurons of the arcuate nucleus

    **D** Inhibition of NPY neurons of the arcuate nucleus

    **E** Inhibition of AgRP neurons of the arcuate nucleus

3. A 50-year-old man has been referred to the cardiology clinic after presenting with worsening exercise tolerance and shortness of breath. On examination, he has a mid-diastolic murmur with a loud S1. Which ECG abnormality is commonly seen in these patients?

    **A** Ventricular pre-excitation

    **B** Atrial fibrillation

    **C** ST elevation

    **D** Prolonged PR interval

    **E** Prolonged QT interval

4. A 43-year-old man with a background of hypothyroidism has presented to his GP complaining of ongoing tiredness and fatigue, despite starting treatment with levothyroxine. Over the last 3 months, he has lost 4 kg in weight. A blood test reveals the following results.

    Na: 122 mmol/L (135–145)
    K: 6.1 mmol/L (3.5–5.0)
    Urea: 4.1 mmol/L (4–7)
    Creatinine: 86 $\mu$mol/L (60–120)
    TSH: 3.4 mU/L (0.4–4.0)
    fT4: 16 pmol/L (12–30)

Given the likely diagnosis, which of the following medications is likely to be used in his treatment?

    **A** Fludrocortisone

    **B** Spironolactone

**C** Liothyronine
**D** Metyrapone
**E** Carbimazole

5. Which symptom is most likely associated with a stroke involving the posterior cerebral artery?

   **A** Inappropriate social behaviour
   **B** Contralateral hemiplegia
   **C** Bitemporal hemianopia
   **D** Expressive aphasia
   **E** Prosopagnosia

6. A 43-year-old woman presents to A&E with colicky right upper quadrant pain and vomiting. She has experienced this pain on several occasions in the past, however, this episode is more intense and has not resolved with time.
   What is the most likely diagnosis?

   **A** Ureteric colic
   **B** Gallstones
   **C** Bowel obstruction
   **D** Hepatitis A
   **E** Peptic ulcer disease

7. A 65-year-old man has been referred to the outpatient orthopaedic clinic by his GP after his knee pain has failed to resolve with weight loss, physiotherapy and simple analgesia. Based on his symptoms, he was diagnosed with osteoarthritis and is being considered for a knee replacement.
   Given the most likely diagnosis, which of the following features are you most likely to see on an X-ray of the affected knee?

   **A** Widening of the joint space
   **B** Bony outgrowths at joint margins
   **C** Soft tissue swelling

    **D** Microfractures of tibial plateau

    **E** Patellar osteosclerosis

8. Which of the following is a direct consequence of damage to type II pneumocytes?

    **A** Alveolar collapse

    **B** Alveolar oedema

    **C** Thickened gas exchange interface

    **D** Fibrin deposition

    **E** Neutrophil recruitment

9. A 36-year-old woman presents to her GP complaining of ongoing fatigue. She finds that she is very tired towards the end of the day despite there being no changes in her activity levels. On examination, she has a smoothly enlarged, non-tender thyroid gland.
   What is the most likely diagnosis?

    **A** De Quervain's thyroiditis

    **B** Hashimoto's thyroiditis

    **C** Graves' disease

    **D** Pituitary adenoma

    **E** Toxic multinodular goitre

10. A 68-year-old man with a background of COPD presents with a 4-day history of worsening shortness of breath and a cough. His chest X-ray reveals widespread emphysematous changes with dense consolidation in the right lower zone. An ABG reveals the following results.

    pH: 7.28 (7.35–7.45)

    $PaO_2$: 6.9 on room air (>10 kPa)

    $PaCO_2$: 7.6 (4.5–6 kPa)

    $HCO_3^-$: 31 (22–26mmol/L)

    What is the most likely diagnosis?

A Partially compensated respiratory acidosis
B Partially compensated metabolic acidosis
C Compensated respiratory acidosis
D Compensated metabolic acidosis
E Type I respiratory failure

11. A 37-year-old woman has been brought in by ambulance after being involved in a high-speed car accident. She is noted to have reduced pin-prick sensation in her right leg and paralysis of the left leg. An MRI scan reveals a vertebral fracture that has caused hemisection of the spinal cord. Regarding the peripheral pain pathways, where do the first-order neurones synapse with second-order neurones?

A Thalamus
B Cuneate nucleus
C Gracile nucleus
D Substantia gelatinosa
E Primary somatosensory cortex

12. A 71-year-old man has been admitted to the cardiology ward after presenting with sudden-onset shortness of breath and a productive cough. A chest X-ray on admission revealed widespread pulmonary oedema that is thought to be secondary to heart failure given his background of ischaemic heart disease. He is started on furosemide, which works by blocking the Na-K-Cl triple transporter.
In which part of the nephron will this drug act?

A Proximal convoluted tubule
B Distal convoluted tubule
C Thin descending limb of loop of Henle
D Thick ascending limb of loop of Henle
E Collecting duct

13. Which of the following is a difference that you would expect to see in a patient with asthma undergoing spirometry testing compared to a patient with COPD?

    **A** Lower FEV1
    **B** Higher FVC
    **C** Bronchodilator reversibility
    **D** Higher pO2
    **E** Lower total lung capacity

14. A 57-year-old woman with a background of stage 5 chronic kidney disease has been admitted to A&E with severe right-sided loin pain. A urine dipstick reveals microscopic haematuria and a CT KUB identifies a urinary tract calculus at the right pelvi-ureteric junction. She mentions that she has been feeling increasingly thirsty over the last 2 months, however, she knows not to drink too much water because of her poor renal function. She receives haemodialysis three times per week. Which of the following can explain her current presentation?

    **A** Inadequate 1α-hydroxylase activity
    **B** Parathyroid gland hyperplasia
    **C** Dietary vitamin D deficiency
    **D** Transitional cell carcinoma
    **E** Renal osteodystrophy

15. A 17-year-old boy is referred to the gastroenterology outpatient clinic after presenting to his GP with a 2-month history of persistent diarrhoea and weight loss. He undergoes an endoscopy to further investigate a possible diagnosis of inflammatory bowel disease.
    Which of the following features is more likely to be seen in ulcerative colitis than Crohn's disease?

    **A** Fistulae
    **B** Skip lesions
    **C** Strictures
    **D** Transmural inflammation
    **E** Rectal involvement

16. A 71-year-old woman has recently been diagnosed with amyotrophic lateral sclerosis after presenting with a 6-month history of worsening

muscle weakness. On examination, she has marked atrophy in her lower limbs with decreased muscle tone. Her plantars are upgoing and her knee jerk reflexes are brisk.
Which of the following is an upper motor neurone sign?

A  Rigidity
B  Muscle atrophy
C  Fibrillations
D  Spasticity
E  Hyporeflexia

17. A 53-year-old woman is brought into A&E with severe chest pain that began 3 hours ago. An ECG reveals ST elevation in leads II, III and aVF.
Which of the following coronary arteries is most likely to be affected?

A  Left anterior descending coronary artery
B  Left circumflex coronary artery
C  Left marginal artery
D  Right coronary artery
E  Posterior descending coronary artery

18. A 39-year-old man has been referred to the gastroenterology clinic after presenting with a 6-month history of worsening swallowing difficulty. On further questioning, he describes the food getting stuck after he swallows. A barium swallow is conducted, and a diagnosis of achalasia is made.
Which of the following best describes the pathophysiology of achalasia?

A  Reflux of stomach acid due to lower oesophageal sphincter incompetence
B  Increased force of peristaltic movements within the oesophagus
C  Failure of relaxation of the lower oesophageal sphincter

    **D** Hypertrophy of the pylorus

    **E** Mass effect within the gastric lumen

19. An oral glucose tolerance test may be used to test for aberrant pituitary secretion of which of the following hormones?

    **A** Cortisol

    **B** Insulin

    **C** Growth hormone

    **D** ACTH

    **E** Thyroxine

20. A 64-year-old man with known lung cancer is being reviewed by acute oncology after developing headaches and double vision. On examination, he has right-sided ptosis with a fixed, dilated pupil with no response to light.

    Which cranial nerve is responsible for the efferent branch of the pupillary light reflex?

    **A** Optic nerve

    **B** Abducens nerve

    **C** Trochlear nerve

    **D** Oculomotor nerve

    **E** Vestibulocochlear nerve

21. A 45-year-old patient with a background of stage 5 chronic kidney disease has been started on dialysis, which she will require three times per week.

    Which of the following electrolyte abnormalities is most likely to occur in this patient as a consequence of her renal disease?

    **A** Hypernatraemia

    **B** Hyperkalaemia

    **C** Hypercalcaemia

    **D** Hypophosphataemia

    **E** Hypoglycaemia

22. Which of the following spirometry parameters would increase in a patient with COPD?

    A  Tidal volume
    B  Expiratory reserve volume
    C  Residual volume
    D  Inspiratory reserve volume
    E  Vital capacity

23. In myocardial infarction, the rupture of an atherosclerotic plaque results in platelet activation and thrombus formation.
    Which of the following factors is directly responsible for the rupture of the fibrous cap of the atherosclerotic plaque?

    A  Oxidised low-density lipoproteins
    B  Matrix metalloproteinases
    C  Reactive oxygen species
    D  Transforming growth factor beta
    E  Platelet-derived growth factor

24. A 58-year-old woman, who has recently had a mastectomy for breast cancer, has been started on letrozole to reduce the risk of recurrence of breast cancer. She underwent menopause at the age of 51 years.
    What is the mechanism of action of this drug?

    A  Oestrogen receptor antagonist
    B  Oestradiol analogue
    C  Aromatase inhibitor
    D  GnRH agonist
    E  $5\alpha$ reductase inhibitor

25. A 34-year-old man has been admitted to the inpatient psychiatry ward under the mental health act after developing paranoid delusions about an evil spirit that was commanding him to kill his wife. On three occasions, he said that he had seen the spirit in his house

in the form of a faceless man. He has been started on olanzapine (antipsychotic) which has brought about a significant improvement in his symptoms.

Which of the following mechanisms would best explain the hallucinations that this patient has been experiencing?

    A  Excess dopamine activity in the mesolimbic system
    B  Insufficient dopamine activity in the basal ganglia
    C  Excess cholinergic activity within the mesocortical system
    D  Insufficient cholinergic activity within the hippocampus
    E  Excess adrenergic activity within the primary visual cortex

26. A 56-year-old woman has presented to her GP complaining of a 6-month history of fatigue. She has a background of hypothyroidism and Addison's disease which have been treated with thyroxine and regular corticosteroids. A panel of blood tests are requested by the GP (results below).

Hb: 101 g/L (115–155)
MCV: 107 fL (82–100)
WCC: $6.1 \times 10^9$/L (4–11)
Neut: $4.5 \times 10^9$/L (2–7)
CRP: 2 mg/L (< 0.6)
B12: 82 pg/mL (190–950)
Folate: 13 ng/mL (2–20)
Serum Iron: 82 $\mu$g/dL (60–170)

Damage to which of the following cell types could explain this clinical scenario?

    A  Chief cell
    B  Enteroendocrine cell
    C  Paneth cell
    D  Enterocyte
    E  Parietal cell

27. An 88-year-old man is reviewed in the neurology clinic after suffering an ischaemic stroke. He is able to understand simple commands and can express himself despite mild dysarthria, however, he is unable to repeat a specific phrase.

    Damage to which part of the brain is likely to be responsible for this neurological manifestation?

    **A** Arcuate fasciculus
    **B** Uncinate fasciculus
    **C** Primary motor cortex
    **D** Broca's area
    **E** Wernicke's area

28. A 41-year-old man has been brought into A&E with sudden-onset shortness of breath and right-sided chest pain. His chest X-ray is normal, however, a CTPA confirms the presence of a clot within the right lower lobe.

    Which of the following is <u>least</u> likely to be used in the initial or long-term treatment of his condition?

    **A** Aspirin
    **B** Warfarin
    **C** Heparin
    **D** Apixaban
    **E** Rivaroxaban

29. A 77-year-old man presents to his GP with a 6-month history of urinary difficulties. He mentions that he has been going to the toilet to urinate over 10 times per day including being woken up at night with an urge to urinate. When he goes to the toilet, he takes quite a long time to establish urinary flow and often does not feel completely empty after voiding. A digital rectal examination is performed during the consultation and a smoothly enlarged prostate gland with a palpable midline sulcus is felt.

    Which part of the prostate gland is most likely to be affected in this patient?

A Peripheral zone
B Central zone
C Transitional zone
D Fibromuscular zone
E Seminal vesicle

30. An 85-year-old man is referred to the medical team after his GP noticed a raised calcium level (3.1 mmol/L) on a recent blood test. On admission, he explains that he has become quite constipated recently and has been urinating increasingly frequently. He has recently been diagnosed with probable lung cancer and is awaiting further investigations.

Which of the following types of lung cancer is most likely?

A Small cell lung cancer
B Squamous cell lung cancer
C Adenocarcinoma
D Large cell lung cancer
E Mesothelioma

# Answers

## 1. D (*Streptococcus pneumoniae*)

Community-acquired pneumonia (CAP) is a common condition, especially amongst the elderly, and it typically presents with a cough, shortness of breath and fever. The most common cause of community-acquired pneumonia is *Streptococcus pneumoniae*. *Haemophilus influenzae* is another common cause. CAP can also be caused by atypical organisms (*Mycoplasma pneumoniae*, *Chlamydia pneumoniae* and *Legionella pneumoniae*) which present with slightly 'atypical' symptoms such as a dry cough, confusion and diarrhoea. The treatment of CAP typically involves the combination of amoxicillin or co-amoxiclav and clarithromycin (to provide atypical cover).

## 2. B (Stimulation of orexigenic neurons of the lateral hypothalamic area)

Leptin is a hormone that is produced by white adipose tissue. It interacts with neuropeptide Y (NPY) and agouti-related peptide (AgRP) orexigenic neurones and POMC anorexigenic neurones within the arcuate nucleus. NPY/AgRP neurones have a stimulatory effect on appetite which acts by stimulating the paraventricular nucleus. This effect is inhibited by leptin. Leptin also stimulates the release of melanocyte-stimulating hormone by POMC neurones in the arcuate nucleus. The melanocyte-stimulating hormone binds to MC4 receptors in the paraventricular nuclei and promotes satiety. In congenital leptin deficiency, a reduction in circulating leptin leads to reduced inhibition of the orexigenic neurones of the lateral hypothalamic area, thereby promoting hunger and food intake.

## 3. B (Atrial fibrillation)

Mitral stenosis refers to narrowing of the mitral valve and it is most commonly caused by rheumatic heart disease. It may lead to symptoms of left heart failure such as shortness of breath, orthopnoea and a productive cough. Mitral valve diseases are commonly associated with atrial fibrillation. It is thought to occur due to the dilation of the left atrium resulting in disruption of the electrical impulses that pass through the atria.

Ventricular pre-excitation occurs in Wolff–Parkinson–White syndrome. The presence of an accessory pathway between the atria and ventricles, known as the bundle of Kent, allows the wave of depolarisation to bypass the atrioventricular node and begin to depolarise the ventricles. This gives rise to a slurred upstroke on the ECG and can lead to supraventricular tachycardia. ST elevation is a feature of myocardial infarction. First-degree heart block causes a fixed, prolonged PR interval. A prolonged QT interval can be congenital or acquired due to electrolyte abnormalities (e.g. hypomagnesemia) or certain medications (e.g. citalopram).

### 4. A (Fludrocortisone)

Primary adrenocortical failure most often occurs due to autoimmune destruction of the adrenal cortex (Addison's disease). It presents insidiously with features such as fatigue, weight loss, low blood pressure and increased skin pigmentation. Blood tests may reveal low sodium and high potassium due to a lack of mineralocorticoid activity. Autoimmune diseases often come hand in hand, so the background of hypothyroidism in this patient is a significant finding. The investigation of primary adrenal insufficiency usually involves a 9 am cortisol level and a short synacthen test. Treatment involves replacing the hormones that the patient's adrenal glands are unable to produce: cortisol (using prednisolone) and aldosterone (using fludrocortisone).

Spironolactone is a mineralocorticoid receptor antagonist that reduces sodium reabsorption in the distal convoluted tubule and collecting duct. It is used as a diuretic in the treatment of heart failure and chronic liver disease with ascites. Liothyronine is a synthetic form of T3. It may be used by specialists in patients who are unable to convert T4 into T3. Metyrapone is an $11\beta$-hydroxylase inhibitor which can inhibit cortisol synthesis. It may be used in the treatment of Cushing syndrome. Carbimazole is a thionamide that inhibits thyroid peroxidase within follicular cells, thereby reducing the synthesis of thyroid hormone. It is used in the treatment of hyperthyroidism.

## 5. E (Prosopagnosia)

The posterior cerebral artery supplies the occipital lobe, which is where the primary visual cortex is located. A stroke involving this artery would likely cause a significant visual field defect (usually homonymous hemianopia with macular sparing), visual agnosia (inability to recognise commonplace objects) and prosopagnosia (inability to recognise faces).

Inappropriate social behaviour is seen in strokes affecting the frontal lobe. Contralateral hemiplegia may occur with anterior or middle cerebral artery strokes which affect the primary motor cortex. Bitemporal hemianopia occurs due to disruption of the optic nerve fibres at the optic chiasm. This may be caused by a pituitary adenoma or craniopharyngioma. Expressive aphasia is the inability to understand written or spoken speech. It occurs due to damage to Broca's area which is found in the frontal lobe.

## 6. B (Gallstones)

Gallstones are accumulations of cholesterol and bile that precipitate within the gallbladder and can cause an obstruction within the biliary tree. It can cause a spectrum of disease ranging from biliary colic to ascending cholangitis. The temporary presence of a stone within the cystic or common bile duct can trigger painful contractions of the bile duct in an attempt to relieve the obstruction. This tends to come on after eating fatty meals because the presence of fatty acids within the duodenum triggers the release of cholecystokinin from enteroendocrine mucosal cells which then promotes gallbladder contraction. Gallstones are common and risk factors include female sex, 40–60 years of age and obesity.

Ureteric colic is caused by the presence of a urinary tract calculus within the kidney or ureter. It causes 'loin to groin' colicky pain. Bowel obstruction causes generalised abdominal pain, abdominal distension and vomiting. Hepatitis A is an acute viral hepatitis that is acquired via the faeco-oral route. It causes jaundice, diarrhoea and vomiting. Peptic ulcer disease is characterised by burning epigastric pain. If it bleeds, it can cause melaena and haematemesis.

## 7. B (Bony outgrowths at joint margins)

Osteoarthritis is a degenerative condition of the joint that results from the breakdown of articular cartilage. Despite the prefix 'osteo', it is primarily a disease of the cartilage that patients tend to develop either due to the presence of fragile articular cartilage (typically in younger patients with a strong family history) or abnormal forces through the joint (typically seen in obesity and sportspeople). The main radiographic features of osteoarthritis can be remembered using the mnemonic **LOSS**: **L**oss of joint space, **O**steophytes (bony spurs at joint margins), **S**ubchondral cysts and **S**ubchondral sclerosis.

## 8. A (Alveolar collapse)

The alveoli are lined by type I and type II pneumocytes. Type I pneumocytes are fewer in number but are thin and account for a greater proportion of the alveolar surface area. Being extremely thin enables them to carry out efficient gas exchange. Type II pneumocytes are responsible for the production of surfactant. Surfactant is a fluid that is rich in phospholipids and proteins and serves the function of reducing alveolar surface tension and preventing the collapse of the alveoli.

## 9. B (Hashimoto's thyroiditis)

Thyroxine, produced by the thyroid gland, is a key determinant of our basal metabolic rate. Hypothyroidism, therefore, results in the general 'slowing down' of various bodily functions. This manifests with a variety of features including fatigue, weight gain, constipation and low mood. The most common cause of hypothyroidism is Hashimoto's thyroiditis — an autoimmune condition characterised by destruction of the thyroid follicular cells. The infiltration of the thyroid gland by lymphocytes results in enlargement and fibrosis.

De Quervain's thyroiditis (also known as viral thyroiditis) is acute inflammation of the thyroid gland caused by viral infection. It begins with an initial hyperthyroid phase during which viral-induced damage to the thyroid gland results in the release of excess amounts of stored thyroxine. This later progresses to a hypothyroid phase in which the stores of thyroxine have been depleted and the synthesis of thyroid hormone from the damaged cells is insufficient to achieve normal concentrations of thyroxine. Eventually, once the thyroid gland recovers, the patient will become euthyroid. Patients with De Quervain's thyroiditis will present with features of hyperthyroidism and viral infection (e.g. fever, tender goitre). Graves' disease is the most common cause of hyperthyroidism. It is an autoimmune disease characterised by the production of TSH-receptor stimulating antibodies. It will cause a smoothly enlarged, non-tender goitre. A pituitary adenoma may potentially cause hyperthyroidism due to excessive production of TSH. Toxic multinodular goitre is a condition in which multiple nodules form within the thyroid gland, some of which can autonomously produce thyroid hormone. It causes hyperthyroidism.

**10. A (Partially compensated respiratory acidosis)**

This patient has presented with an infective exacerbation of COPD. When approaching ABGs, it is important to remember that there are two main determinants of pH: carbon dioxide (regulated by the lungs) and bicarbonate (regulated by the kidneys). First and foremost, the pH determines whether the patient is acidotic or alkalotic. If a patient is acidotic (as in this case), proceed to check the carbon dioxide concentration. If raised, it is suggestive of a respiratory acidosis. If low, it is suggestive of respiratory compensation for a metabolic acidosis. The bicarbonate can give an indication of whether the patient is a chronic carbon dioxide retainer. Some patients with COPD may have a chronically elevated carbon dioxide level. This results in increased retention of bicarbonate by the kidneys in order to maintain a normal blood pH. In this case, the patient has a high bicarbonate level suggesting that the patient is trying to compensate, however, as the pH is still low, it is described as 'partial compensation'. This patient also has type II respiratory failure which is defined by a $PaCO_2 > 6$ kPa and a $PaO^2 < 8$ kPa.

### 11. D (Substantia gelatinosa)

The spinothalamic tract is a sensory pathway that is responsible for conveying crude, pain and temperature sensation from the peripheries. It differs from the pathways for fine touch and proprioception as it decussates and synapses at the level at which the first-order neurone enters the spinal cord. The synapse between the first- and second-order neurones is found within an area of the spinal cord called the substantia gelatinosa. The second-order neurone will then ascend through the spinal and synapse with third-order neurones within the thalamus. The third-order neurones will then terminate at the primary somatosensory cortex.

### 12. D (Thick ascending limb of loop of Henle)

Loop diuretics, such as furosemide and bumetanide, are medications that are commonly used to treat fluid overload (e.g. in acute heart failure). They work by blocking the Na-K-Cl triple transporter in the thick ascending limb of the loop of Henle, thereby preventing sodium reabsorption. The ensuing high concentration of sodium within the tubule will draw water into the tubule thereby increasing urine output.

### 13. C (Bronchodilator reversibility)

Spirometry may be used in the investigation of patients with COPD and asthma. They are both common obstructive lung diseases and may yield relatively similar results on spirometry testing. Both are associated with a decrease in FEV1 (forced expiratory volume in 1 second) and FVC (forced vital capacity). The decrease in FEV1 usually exceeds that of FVC thereby resulting in a decrease in the FEV1/FVC ratio. Obstructive airways diseases are characterised by an FEV1/FVC ratio < 0.7. The main difference between asthma and COPD is that the airway obstruction in asthma can be reversed with the use of a bronchodilator.

### 14. B (Parathyroid gland hyperplasia)

Patients with chronic kidney disease tend to, initially, become hypocalcaemic because of inadequate 1α-hydroxylase activity within the kidneys.

The activation of vitamin D occurs in two stages. Firstly, vitamin D is converted in the liver by 25-hydroxylase to 25-hydroxy vitamin D. This then travels to the kidneys where 1α-hydroxylase converts it to the active form of vitamin D, 1,25-dihydroxy vitamin D (also known as calcitriol). The inability to activate vitamin D in chronic kidney disease results in hypocalcaemia. In response, the parathyroid gland will begin to produce increasing amounts of parathyroid hormone (PTH). This is known as secondary hyperparathyroidism. Prolonged stimulation of PTH release from the parathyroid gland results in parathyroid hyperplasia, which can eventually start producing PTH independent of the feedback from serum calcium. This is known as tertiary hyperparathyroidism. The ensuing hypercalcaemia presents with a variety of symptoms including bone pain, kidney stones, polyuria and polydipsia.

Inadequate 1α-hydroxylase activity results in a deficiency of activated vitamin D which, in turn, results in secondary hyperparathyroidism. Dietary vitamin D deficiency would cause hypocalcaemia. Transitional cell carcinoma is less likely to cause hypercalcaemia than tertiary hyperparathyroidism. Renal osteodystrophy refers to the spectrum of bone diseases that result from poor renal function in patients with chronic kidney disease.

## 15. E (Rectal involvement)

Inflammatory bowel disease is an umbrella term that encompasses two diseases — Crohn's disease and ulcerative colitis. They present relatively similarly — with chronic diarrhoea, weight loss and, sometimes, rectal bleeding — however, they have some key differences in their pathophysiology and disease patterns. Ulcerative colitis, as the word 'colitis' suggests, only affects the colon. The inflammation begins in the rectum and spreads proximally in a continuous manner. Furthermore, the inflammation is superficial and only affects the mucosa. In Crohn's disease, the inflammation can occur at any point from mouth to anus and it is discontinuous, meaning that the inflammation can occur in patches. The inflammation is transmural, and it has a predilection for affecting the terminal ileum. Furthermore, Crohn's disease is more strongly associated with causing various anatomical complications such as strictures and fistulae.

### 16. D (Spasticity)

Motor neurone disease is a neurodegenerative disorder characterised by the progressive destruction of motor neurones. There are several subtypes of motor neurone disease of which amyotrophic lateral sclerosis is the most common. It can cause a mixture of upper and lower motor neurone signs. Examples of upper motor neurone signs include spasticity, hyper-reflexia, clonus and upgoing plantars. It is thought to occur due to the disruption of descending inhibitory tracts that normally moderate tone and movements. Examples of lower motor neurone signs include hypotonia, hyporeflexia, absent reflexes, fasciculations and fibrillations. Rigidity is another term used to describe increased muscle tone; however, it is mainly used in the context of Parkinson's disease. Rigidity refers to increased tone in all directions of joint movement with no velocity-dependence. Spasticity, on the other hand, is an upper motor neurone sign that is both velocity- and direction-dependent.

### 17. D (Right coronary artery)

The leads in which ST elevation is seen, in the context of chest pain, can indicate which aspect of the heart and, hence, which coronary artery is affected.

| ST elevation in leads | Type of MI | Coronary artery involved |
|---|---|---|
| V1, V2, V3, V4 | Anterior | Left anterior descending |
| I, aVL, V5, V6 | Lateral | Left circumflex |
| II, III, aVF | Inferior | Right coronary artery |

### 18. C (Failure of relaxation of the lower oesophageal sphincter)

Achalasia is a condition that causes dysphagia due to failure of relaxation of the lower oesophageal sphincter. It results from the absence of ganglion cells within Auerbach's plexus in the wall of the lower oesophagus. Swallowed food may get stuck in the lower oesophagus, causing dysphagia and vomiting. A barium swallow may reveal oesophageal dilatation that is sometimes described as having a 'bird's beak' appearance. To treat achalasia, pneumatic dilation or surgery may be considered.

## 19. C (Growth hormone)

Acromegaly is a condition that arises due to excessive production of growth hormone from the pituitary gland. It may present insidiously with changes in physical appearance such as prominent supraorbital ridges and an increase in hand and foot size. The main diagnostic investigations for acromegaly include measuring serum IGF-I levels (elevated in acromegaly) and conducting an oral glucose tolerance test. The administration of glucose, under normal conditions, would result in a decrease in pituitary growth hormone release, however, in acromegaly, there is a paradoxical rise in growth hormone. A pituitary MRI scan may also be used to visualise a pituitary tumour that is causing acromegaly.

## 20. D (Oculomotor nerve)

Light entering the pupil will strike the photoreceptors of the retina which create an electrical impulse that passes along fibres of the optic nerve that project towards the pretectal nucleus of the midbrain. A second-order neurone then projects from the pretectal nucleus towards the right and left Edinger–Westphal nuclei. Then, parasympathetic fibres of the oculomotor nerve project from the Edinger–Westphal nucleus towards the ciliary ganglion. Finally, the short posterior ciliary nerve innervates the pupillary sphincter and causes miosis. The oculomotor nerve is also responsible for providing motor innervation of the levator palpebrae superioris and several extraocular muscles. Oculomotor nerve palsy, therefore, may cause the eye to be depressed and abducted, with ptosis and mydriasis. The optic nerve transmits electrical impulses from the retina towards the primary visual cortex. It is responsible for the afferent branch of the pupillary light reflex. The abducens nerve innervates the lateral rectus and is responsible for abduction of the eye. The trochlear nerve innervates the superior oblique which is responsible for internal rotation and depression of the eye. The vestibulocochlear nerve is important in hearing and balance.

## 21. B (Hyperkalaemia)

Chronic kidney disease (CKD) is defined as a decrease in glomerular filtration rate of less than 60 mL/min/$1.73m^2$ over the course of 3 months or more. It is most commonly caused by hypertension and diabetes mellitus. The main functions of the kidney include fluid and electrolyte homeostasis, acid-base balance, toxin and waste excretion, and hormone production (erythropoietin and $1\alpha$-hydroxylase). Therefore, the consequences of CKD occur as a result of a loss of the aforementioned functions. The net effect of the kidneys on electrolytes is to reabsorb sodium and bicarbonate and excrete potassium and protons. Therefore, an impairment in kidney function (as seen in CKD) will result in hyponatraemia, acidosis and hyperkalaemia.

## 22. C (Residual volume)

Residual volume is defined as the volume of air within the lungs that persists upon maximal exhalation. In patients with COPD, their airways are narrowed and fragile meaning that they are susceptible to collapse during exhalation. This means that air gets trapped within the alveoli during exhalation and, hence, does not participate in gas exchange. This results in an increase in residual volume.

## 23. B (Matrix metalloproteinases)

The process of atherosclerosis begins with the passage of low-density lipoproteins (LDLs) through the endothelium into the subendothelial space of the coronary arteries. Subsequently, macrophages transmigrate into the subendothelial space and release reactive oxygen species. LDLs become oxidised and are, subsequently, detected by scavenger receptors and phagocytosed by macrophages. The accumulation of cholesterol crystals within the macrophages turns them into lipid-filled foam cells, which will eventually die and form a necrotic lipid core within the atheroma. Matrix metalloproteinases are enzymes that break down extracellular matrix proteins. In the case of atherosclerosis, matrix metalloproteinases can hydrolyse the collagen fibres of the fibrous cap resulting in rupture and exposure of the pro-thrombotic subendothelial material.

## 24. C (Aromatase inhibitor)

Breast cancers are often described by the presence of certain hormone receptors on the surface of the tumour cells. Many breast cancers will have oestrogen receptors and their growth will be stimulated by oestrogen. Therefore, hormonal treatment of breast cancer aims to block this harmful effect of oestrogen. This can be achieved using selective oestrogen receptors modulators, such as tamoxifen, which have anti-oestrogenic effects in the breast. In postmenopausal women, oestrogen is primarily produced via the peripheral conversion of various precursors (e.g. testosterone) in adipose tissue by the action of aromatase. Letrozole is an aromatase inhibitor that reduces the production of oestrogen from precursors.

## 25. A (Excess dopamine activity in the mesolimbic system)

Psychosis is defined as a loss of contact with reality, which may manifest with delusions (false, fixed beliefs which are held despite evidence to disprove them) and hallucinations (false visual perceptions). Schizophrenia is a chronic condition in which patients develop an array of behavioural and psychological symptoms such as social withdrawal, delusions and hallucinations. These symptoms may be categorised as positive symptoms (e.g. delusions and hallucinations) and negative symptoms (e.g. social withdrawal). The positive symptoms are thought to arise due to excessive dopaminergic activity within the mesolimbic system. This is why the mainstay of treatment of psychotic conditions involves dopamine antagonists (e.g. olanzapine).

## 26. E (Parietal cell)

Pernicious anaemia is an autoimmune condition characterised by immune-mediated damage to gastric parietal cells resulting in reduced intrinsic factor production. Intrinsic factor is required for the protection of vitamin B12 as it transits from the stomach to the terminal ileum where it is absorbed. The lack of intrinsic factor in pernicious anaemia therefore results in vitamin B12 deficiency. As it is an autoimmune disease, it is more likely to arise in patients who have a background of other autoimmune diseases such as thyroid disease and Addison's disease.

Vitamin B12 is an important component in the production of DNA nucleotides, so deficiency results in insufficient red cell production (leading to megaloblastic anaemia) and insufficient myelin production (leading to neurological manifestation such as peripheral neuropathy).

Chief cells are found within the stomach and are primarily responsible for producing pepsinogen which gets activated to pepsin. Enteroendocrine G-cells are located around the pyloric sphincter and are responsible for releasing gastrin which stimulates gastric acid secretion. Paneth cells within the lining of the small intestine will produce antimicrobial enzymes that regulate the gut microbiome. Enterocytes are the cells that line the intestines and are responsible for absorption of various nutrients.

### 27. A (Arcuate fasciculus)

Wernicke's and Broca's areas are parts of the brain that are responsible for language comprehension and speech generation, respectively. Damage to Wernicke's area would result in an inability to understand written or spoken language (receptive aphasia) and damage to Broca's area would result in an inability to produce coherent, sensical speech (expressive aphasia). The arcuate fasciculus is the white matter tract that links these two areas. Damage to the arcuate fasciculus would result in an inability to repeat speech (conduction aphasia).

### 28. A (Aspirin)

It is important to avoid getting confused between antiplatelets and anticoagulants as the circumstances in which they are used differ. Virchow's triad denotes the three main factors that contribute towards blood clot formation: vessel wall injury, stasis and hypercoagulability. In the case of a deep vein thrombosis, pulmonary embolism or atrial fibrillation, clots form due to stasis resulting in an increased risk of coagulation factor activation and, hence, thrombus formation. Therefore, in these circumstances anticoagulants (e.g. apixaban, warfarin, heparin) are used. In the case of myocardial infarction or strokes due to carotid atherosclerosis, clots form due to atherosclerotic plaque rupture and platelet activation. Therefore, antiplatelets (e.g. aspirin, clopidogrel) are used.

### 29.  C (Transitional zone)

Benign prostatic hyperplasia (BPH) is a common condition in middle-aged and elderly men which presents with lower urinary tract symptoms (frequency, urgency, nocturia, hesitancy, poor stream, terminal dribbling). It is caused by hyperplasia of the transitional zone of the prostate gland. This part of the prostate gland encircles the prostatic part of the urethra and, hence, enlargement of this part of the prostate gland results in urinary outflow obstruction. BPH may be treated with medications such as alpha blockers (which relax the smooth muscle surrounding the urethra) and 5α-reductase inhibitors (which reduce the conversion of testosterone to dihydrotestosterone).

### 30.  B (Squamous cell lung cancer)

Lung cancers can cause certain paraneoplastic syndromes due to the ectopic expression of various hormones. Squamous cell carcinoma of the lung can express PTHrP (parathyroid hormone-related peptide) which mimics the action of PTH and can lead to hypercalcaemia. Small cell lung cancer has a predilection for producing ectopic ACTH and ADH which can result in Cushing syndrome and SIADH respectively. Small cell lung cancer can also cause Lambert-Eaton syndrome, which is characterised by immune-mediated destruction of the voltage-gated calcium channels resulting in muscle weakness.

# Index

Printed in the United States
by Baker & Taylor Publisher Services